W9-CTJ-001

TOP TRAILS™

Glacier National Park

MUST-DO HIKES FOR EVERYONE

Written by

Jean Arthur

 WILDERNESS PRESS . . . *on the trail since 1967*

Top Trails Glacier National Park: Must-Do Hikes for Everyone
First edition 2014

Copyright © 2014 by Jean Arthur
Front cover photos and interior photos: Jean Arthur
Maps and elevation profiles: Scott McGrew
Cover design: Frances Baca Design and Scott McGrew
Text design: Frances Baca Design
Editor: Holly Cross
Indexer: Rich Carlson

Manufactured in the United States of America

Library of Congress Cataloging-in-Publication Data

Arthur, Jean, 1960-
  Glacier National Park : must-do hikes for everyone / written by Jean Arthur. — 1st edition.
    pages cm. — (Top trails series)
  Includes bibliographical references and index.
  ISBN 978-0-89997-734-8 (alk. paper) — ISBN 0-89997-734-0 (alk. paper) —
   ISBN 978-0-89997-735-5 (ebook); ISBN 978-0-89997-943-4 (hardcover)
  1. Hiking—Montana—Glacier National Park—Guidebooks. 2. Trails—Montana—Glacier
National Park—Guidebooks. 3. Glacier National Park (Mont.)—Guidebooks. I. Title.
  GV199.42.M92G5625 2014
  796.5109786'52—dc23

                        2014015745

Published by: **Wilderness Press**
               An imprint of AdventureKEEN
               2204 First Avenue South, Suite 102
               Birmingham, AL 35233
               800-443-7227
               info@wildernesspress.com
               wildernesspress.com

Visit our website for a complete listing of our books and for ordering information.
Distributed by Publishers Group West

Cover photo: Grinnell Glacier Trail (Trail 36) leads to three glaciers; mountain goats thrive
on the steep slopes of Glacier National Park.

Safety Notice: Although Keen Communications/Wilderness Press and the author have
made every attempt to ensure that the information in this book is accurate at press time,
they are not responsible for any loss, damage, injury, or inconvenience that may occur to
anyone while using this book. You are responsible for your own safety and health while in
the wilderness. The fact that a trail is described in this book does not mean that it will be
safe for you. Be aware that trail conditions can change from day to day. Always check local
conditions, know your own limitations, and consult a map and compass.

The Top Trails™ Series

Wilderness Press

When Wilderness Press published *Sierra North* in 1967, no other trail guide like it existed for the Sierra backcountry. The first run sold out in less than two months, and its success heralded the beginning of Wilderness Press. Since our founding, we have expanded our territories to cover California, Alaska, Hawaii, the US Southwest, the Pacific Northwest, New England, Canada, and the Southeast.

Wilderness Press continues to publish comprehensive, accurate, and readable outdoor books. Hikers, backpackers, kayakers, skiers, snowshoers, climbers, cyclists, and trail runners rely on Wilderness Press for accurate outdoor adventure information.

Top Trails

In its Top Trails guides, Wilderness Press has paid special attention to organization so that you can find the perfect hike each and every time. Whether you're looking for a steep trail to test yourself or a gentle walk in the park, a romantic waterfall or a lakeside view, Top Trails will lead you there.

Each Top Trails guide contains routes for everyone. The trails selected provide a sampling of the very best that the region has to offer. These are the must-do hikes with every feature of the area represented.

Every book in the Top Trails series offers:

- The Wilderness Press commitment to accuracy and reliability
- Ratings and rankings for each trail
- Distances and approximate times
- Easy-to-follow trail notes
- Map and permit information

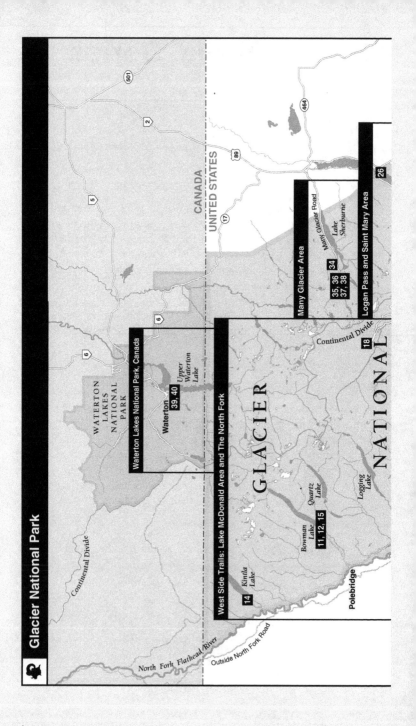

Glacier National Park

Continental Divide

501

2

5

6

6

17

89

464

CANADA

UNITED STATES

WATERTON
LAKES
NATIONAL
PARK

Waterton Lakes National Park, Canada

Waterton

39, 40

Upper Waterton Lake

Many Glacier Area

Many Glacier Road

34

Lake Sherburne

35, 36 37, 38

Logan Pass and Saint Mary Area

26

West Side Trails: Lake McDonald Area and The North Fork

GLACIER

Continental Divide

18

NATIONAL

Kintla Lake

14

Bowman Lake

Quartz Lake

11, 12, 15

Logging Lake

Polebridge

North Fork Flathead River

Outside North Fork Road

Continental Divide

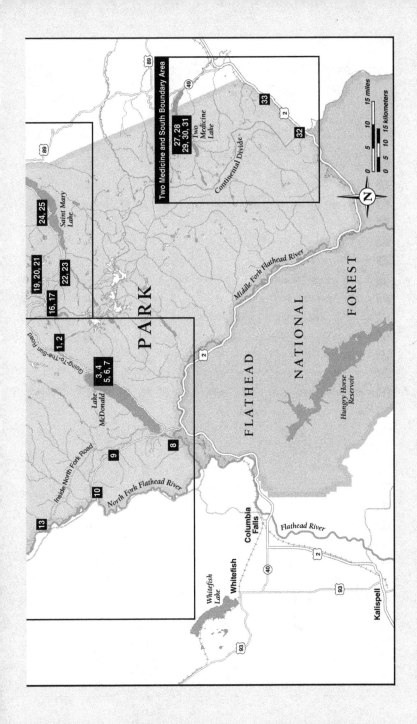

Two Medicine and South Boundary Area

27, 28
29, 30, 31

Two
Medicine
Lake

33

32

Continental Divide

Saint Mary
Lake

24, 25

19, 20, 21

22, 23

16, 17

Going-To-The-Sun Road

1, 2

3, 4
5, 6, 7

Lake
McDonald

PARK

Middle Fork Flathead River

FLATHEAD

NATIONAL

FOREST

Hungry Horse
Reservoir

8

9

Inside North Fork Road

10

13

North Fork Flathead River

Columbia
Falls

Flathead River

Whitefish
Lake

Whitefish

Kalispell

15 miles

15 kilometers

N

TRAIL FEATURES TABLE

Glacier National Park Trails

TRAIL NUMBER AND NAME	Page	Difficulty -12345+	Length in Miles	Type	Day Hiking	Backpacking	Horses	Child-Friendly	Ski/Snowshoe	Wheelchair Access
1. West Side Trails: Lake McDonald Area and the North Fork										
1 Trail of the Cedars	33	1	0.95	Loop	Day Hiking			Child-Friendly		Wheelchair Access
2 Avalanche Lake Trail	37	2	5.8	Out-and-back	Day Hiking			Child-Friendly		
3 Sperry Chalet via Gunsight Pass Trail	41	4	12.4	Out-and-back	Day Hiking	Backpacking	Horses			
4 Snyder Lake Trail	47	3	8.4	Out-and-back	Day Hiking		Horses	Child-Friendly		
5 Fish Lake via Snyder Ridge Fire Trail	53	2	5.8	Out-and-back	Day Hiking			Child-Friendly		
6 Mount Brown Lookout Trail	57	5	10.1	Out-and-back	Day Hiking					
7 Going-to-the-Sun (Winter Trail)	63	1–3	16.8	Out-and-back				Child-Friendly	Ski/Snowshoe	
8 Apgar Lookout Trail	69	3	7.2	Out-and-back	Day Hiking			Child-Friendly		
9 Huckleberry Mountain Lookout Trail	73	3	12.0	Out-and-back	Day Hiking					
10 Forest and Fire Nature Trail	79	1	1.0	Loop	Day Hiking			Child-Friendly		
11 Akokala Lake Trail	83	3	11.6	Out-and-back	Day Hiking	Backpacking		Child-Friendly		
12 Quartz Lake Loop	89	3–4	12.9	Loop	Day Hiking	Backpacking				
13 Logging Lake Trail	93	2	11.0	Out-and-back	Day Hiking	Backpacking		Child-Friendly		
14 Boulder Pass Trail to Hole in the Wall	99	5	40.0	Out-and-back		Backpacking				
15 Bowman Lake Trail to Goat Haunt and Waterton, Canada	105	5	22.3	Point-to-point		Backpacking				
2. Logan Pass and Saint Mary Area										
16 Hidden Lake Trail	123	2	5.14	Out-and-back	Day Hiking			Child-Friendly		
17 Highline Trail to Granite Park Chalet	127	2–3	15.2	Out-and-back	Day Hiking			Child-Friendly		
18 Loop Trail to Granite Park Chalet	133	4	8.4	Out-and-back	Day Hiking			Child-Friendly		
19 Siyeh Bend Trail and Piegan Pass Trail	137	2	2.5	Point-to-point	Day Hiking			Child-Friendly		
20 Siyeh Pass Trail	143	4–5	10.3	Point-to-point	Day Hiking					
21 Piegan Pass Trail	147	3	9.0	Out-and-back	Day Hiking					

USES & ACCESS	TYPE	TERRAIN	FLORA & FAUNA	OTHER
Day Hiking	Loop	Lake	Flora	Secluded
Backpacking	Balloon	Waterfall	Birds	Swimming
Horses	Out-and-back	Glacier	Wildlife	Fishing
Child-Friendly	Point-to-point		Wildfire Ecology	Views
Ski/Snowshoe	DIFFICULTY			Photo Opportunity
Wheelchair Access	-12345+ less more			Geologic Interest
				Historic Interest

| | TERRAIN | | | FLORA & FAUNA | | | | | | | OTHER | | | |
Lake	Waterfall	Glacier	Flora	Birds	Wildlife	Wildfire Ecology	Secluded	Swimming	Fishing	Views	Photo Opportunity	Geologic Interest	Historic Interest
			●	●	●		●			●			
●			●		●							●	
			●		●		●					●	●
●			●		●		●	●	●	●			
●			●		●		●		●			●	●
			●		●		●			●		●	●
			●		●		●			●		●	●
			●	●	●		●			●	●	●	●
			●		●		●			●		●	●
			●	●	●		●					●	●
●			●		●	●	●		●	●		●	●
●			●	●	●	●	●		●			●	●
●			●	●	●		●					●	●
●	●		●		●		●		●	●		●	●
●	●		●	●	●		●					●	●
●			●		●							●	●
			●		●		●			●		●	●
			●			●	●			●	●	●	●
			●	●	●		●			●		●	●
			●	●	●		●			●		●	●
		●	●		●		●					●	●

TRAIL FEATURES TABLE

Glacier National Park Trails

TRAIL NUMBER AND NAME	Page	Difficulty 1-2345+	Length in Miles	Type	Day Hiking	Backpacking	Horses	Chld. Friendly	Ski/Snowshoe	Wheelchair Access
2. Logan Pass and Saint Mary Area (cont'd)										
22 Gunsight Pass Trail to Gunsight Lake	153	3–4	12.6	↗	🚶	🎒				
23 Sun Point Nature Trail to Reynolds Creek	157	2–3	4.5	↘	🚶			👫		
24 Saint Mary Falls Trail	163	2	5.0	↗	🚶			👫		
25 Otokomi Lake/Rose Creek Trail	167	3	10.5	↗	🚶			👫		
26 Beaver Pond Trail	173	1	3.5	↺	🚶			👫		
3. Two Medicine and South Boundary Area										
27 Running Eagle Falls Nature Trail	189	1	0.6	↺	🚶			👫		♿
28 Upper Two Medicine Lake Trail and Twin Falls	193	2–3	4.4–7.6	↺	🚶	🎒				
29 Dawson Pass and Pitamakan Pass Trail	197	5	15.9–17.6	↺	🚶	🎒				
30 Cobalt Lake via Two Medicine Pass Trail	203	3	11.14	↗	🚶	🎒				
31 Mount Henry Trail to Scenic Point	209	4	7.6–12.66	↗	🚶		🐎			
32 Autumn Creek Trail	213	4	5.8	↘					🥾	
33 Firebrand Pass Trail	219	4	10.26–16.0	↗	🚶					
4. Many Glacier Area										
34 Apikuni Falls Trail	235	2	1.8	↗	🚶			👫		
35 Swiftcurrent Lake Nature Trail	239	2	2.6	↺	🚶			👫		
36 Grinnell Glacier Trail	245	3–4	10.2	↗	🚶			👫		
37 Iceberg Lake	249	3	9.6	↗	🚶			👫		
38 Ptarmigan Tunnel Trail	255	3–4	10.5	↗	🚶					
5. Waterton Lakes National Park, Canada										
39 Bertha Lake Trail	269	3	7.0	↗	🚶	🎒		👫		
40 Crypt Lake Trail	273	4	10.9	↗	🚶					

TRAIL FEATURES TABLE

	TERRAIN			FLORA & FAUNA				OTHER						
Lake	Waterfall	Glacier	Flora	Birds	Wildlife	Wildfire Ecology	Secluded	Swimming	Fishing	Views	Photo Opportunity	Geologic Interest	Historic Interest	
X	X	X	X		X		X		X				X	X
X	X		X	X	X		X						X	X
	X		X		X		X						X	
X			X	X	X		X		X		X	X	X	X
			X	X	X		X						X	X
	X		X		X		X		X					
X			X	X	X		X		X		X		X	
X			X		X		X		X		X		X	X
X	X		X		X		X		X				X	X
			X		X		X				X			X
			X		X		X						X	X
			X	X	X		X						X	X
	X	X	X		X		X						X	X
X			X		X		X				X		X	X
X	X	X	X	X	X		X		X				X	X
X			X	X	X		X				X	X	X	
X	X		X		X		X		X				X	X
X	X		X		X		X		X		X		X	X
X	X		X		X		X		X				X	X

Contents

CHAPTER 1

West Side Trails: Lake McDonald Area and the North Fork 21

Map Legend

Featured trail ———————	Bench ⌐	Overlook ◭
Alternate trail -----------------	Boat launch ⛵	Parking 🅿
Freeway ══════════	Bridge ✕	Peak ▲
Highway ═══════════	Campground ▲	Picnic area 🛆
Road —————————	Feature ●	Primitive campsite △
Unpaved road ------------------	Gate ●—●	Ranger station/park office 🏠
Railroad +++++++++++	Glacier ◯	Scenic view ⛰
Continental divide ———————	Golf course 🏌	Trailhead 🚶
Borderline —·—·—·—·—	Lodging ⛏	Travel direction ⇄
Forest/park ▨	Marina ⚓	Waterfall \\
Indian reservation ▨	Outhouse 🏛	Wheelchair access ♿
Water body 〰		
River/stream 〰		
Intermittent stream ------		

Using Top Trails™

Organization of Top Trails

Top Trails is designed to make identifying the perfect trail easy and enjoyable, and to make every outing a success and a pleasure. With this book, you'll discover it's a snap to find the right trail, whether you're planning a major hike or a sociable stroll with friends.

The Region

At the front of this book is the Glacier National Park Area Map (pages iv–v), displaying the entire area covered by this guide and providing a geographic overview. The map is clearly marked to show which area each chapter covers.

The following Glacier National Park Trails Table (pages vi–ix) lists every trail covered in the guide, along with important attributes of each trip.

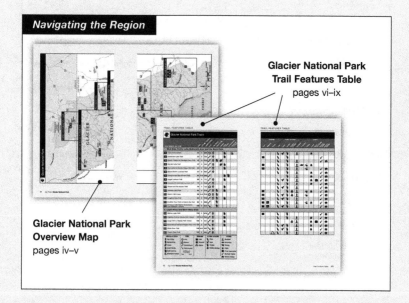

Navigating the Region

Glacier National Park Trail Features Table
pages vi–ix

Glacier National Park Overview Map
pages iv–v

Here you'll find a concise description, basic information, and highlighted features, all indispensable when planning an outing. A quick reading of the Regional Map and the Master Trail Table will provide an overview of the entire region covered by the book.

The Areas

The region covered by this book is divided into five areas, with each chapter corresponding to one area. Each area introduction contains information to help you choose and enjoy a great trail every time out. To find the perfect trip, use the table of contents or the regional map to identify your area of interest, and then turn to the area chapter to find the following:

- An overview of the area, including permit and map information
- An area map with all featured trails clearly marked
- A trail feature table providing trail-by-trail details
- Short trail summaries, written in an informative and accessible style

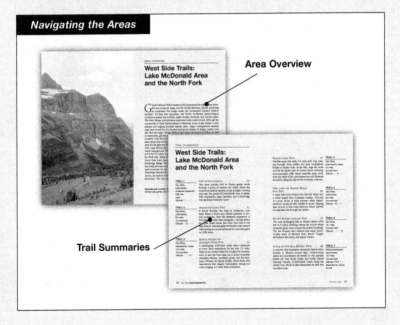

Navigating the Areas

West Side Trails: Lake McDonald Area and the North Fork

Area Overview

Trail Summaries

The Trails

The basic building block of the Top Trails guide is the trail entry. Each one is arranged to make finding and following the trail as simple as possible, with all pertinent information presented in this easy-to-follow format:

- A detailed trail map
- Trail descriptions covering difficulty, length, GPS coordinates, and other essential data
- A written trail text
- Trail milestones providing easy-to-follow, turn-by-turn trail directions

Many trail descriptions offer additional information:

- An elevation profile
- Trail options
- Trail highlights

In the margins of the trail entries, look for icons that point out notable features, such as viewpoints, waterfalls, and wildlife-viewing locations at specific points along the trail.

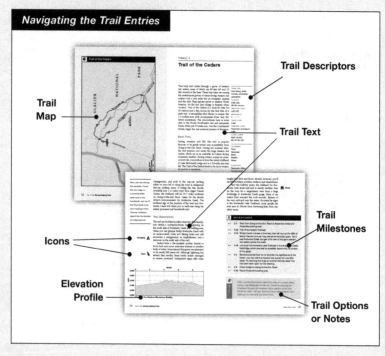

Navigating the Trail Entries

Trail Map

Trail Descriptors

Trail Text

Trail Milestones

Icons

Elevation Profile

Trail Options or Notes

Choosing a Trail

Top Trails provides several ways of choosing a trail, all presented in easy-to-read tables, charts, and maps.

Location

If you know in general where you want to hike, Top Trails makes it easy to find the right trail in the right place. Each chapter begins with a large-scale map showing the starting point of every trail in that area.

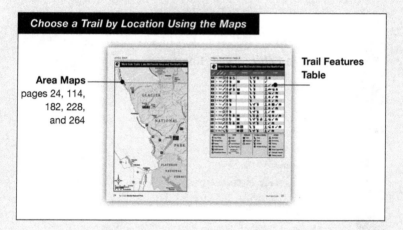

Choose a Trail by Location Using the Maps

Area Maps
pages 24, 114, 182, 228, and 264

Trail Features Table

Features

This guide describes the Top Trails of Glacier National Park and Waterton Lakes National Park, and each trail is chosen because it offers one or more features that make it appealing. Using the trail descriptors, summaries, and tables, you can quickly examine all the trails for the features they offer or seek a particular feature among the list of trails.

Season & Condition

Time of year and current conditions can be important factors in selecting the best trail. For example, an exposed high-elevation trail may be covered in mud and snow in late spring and be a riot of color in midsummer. Where relevant, Top Trails identifies the best and worst conditions for the trails you plan to hike.

Difficulty

Every trail has an overall difficulty rating on a scale of 1 to 5, which takes into consideration factors such as length, elevation change, exposure, trail quality, and season to create one (admittedly subjective) rating.

The ratings assume you are an able-bodied adult in reasonably good shape, using the trail for hiking. The ratings also assume clear and dry weather conditions, although it must be noted that mountain storms can blow in any day of the year, as can snow, hail, and lightning storms.

Readers should make an honest assessment of their own abilities and adjust time estimates accordingly. Also, rain, snow, heat, wind, and poor visibility can all affect the pace on even the easiest of trails.

Top Trails Difficulty Ratings

1 A short trail, generally level, which can typically be completed in 1 hour or less.

2 A route of 1–3 miles, with some up and down, which can be completed in 1–2 hours.

3 A longer route, up to 5 or 6 miles, with some significant uphill and/or downhill sections.

4 A long or steep route, usually more than 5 miles, or with climbs of more than 1,000 vertical feet.

5 The most severe routes, both long and steep, more than 5 miles long and with climbs of 2,500 or more vertical feet. A few longer trails in this range may require backpacking.

Vertical Feet

Every trail entry contains the approximate trail length and the overall elevation gain and loss over the course of the trail. It's important to use both figures when considering a hike. On average, plan 1 hour of hiking for every 2 miles, and add an hour for every 1,000 feet you climb.

The importance of elevation gains is often underestimated by hikers when gauging the difficulty of a trail. The Top Trails measurement accounts for *all* elevation changes, not simply the difference between the highest and lowest points, so that rolling terrain with lots of ups and downs will be identifiable.

The calculation of vertical feet in the Top Trails books is accomplished by a combination of trail measurement and computer-aided estimation. For routes that begin and end at the same spot—loop or out-and-back—the vertical gain exactly matches the vertical descent. With a point-to-point route, the vertical gain and loss will most likely differ, and both figures will be provided in the text.

Finally, for all trail entries, an elevation profile allows you to visualize the topography of the route. These graphics depict the elevation throughout the length of the trail.

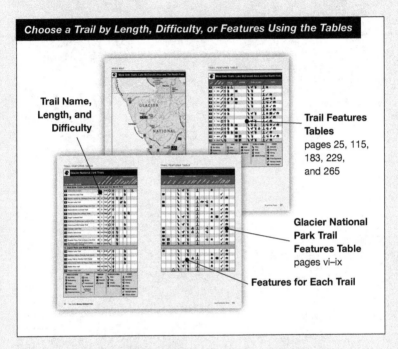

Surface Type

Every trail entry describes the surface of the trail. This information is useful in determining what type of footwear is appropriate. Surface type should also be considered when checking the weather—on a rainy or snowy day early or late in the hiking season, a dirt or rock surface can be a muddy slog; a boardwalk jaunt or a gravel saunter might be a better choice.

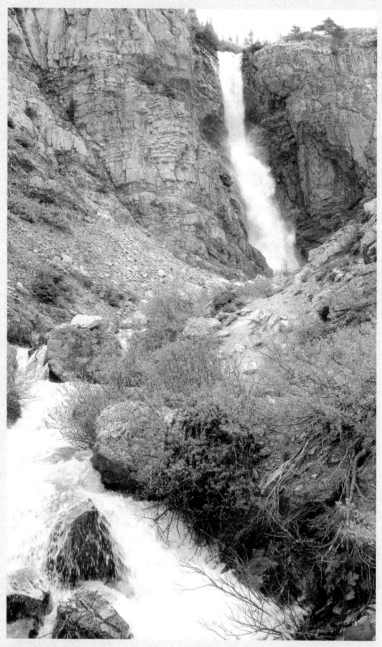

Apikuni Falls Trail *in the Many Glacier Valley provides views of glaciers from points along the short, steep jaunt to the falls.*

Introduction to Glacier National Park and Waterton Lakes National Park

Glacier National Park and Waterton Lakes National Park not only share an international boundary between Montana, USA, and both British Columbia and Alberta, Canada, but the two parks also share a beautiful, unique, and rugged Northern Rockies ecosystem and nearly all the native wildlife that resided here prior to European explorers' visits. The vast ecosystem includes a 10-million-acre wild region with few roads and even fewer human residents. Glacier's 1.2 million acres are rife with waterfalls, lakes, 10,000-foot peaks, and nearly two dozen remaining glaciers. Waterton Lakes' 124,788 acres are where the mountains meet the prairies. It's here in the Crown of the Continent that ecosystems from north, east, south, and west collide at the Rocky Mountains' narrowest point. Distinct is the mingling of ecosystems. The wet Pacific Northwest greets the northern alpine forests, which mix into the prairie-scape. Unique are the multiple watersheds surging from the parks. From the continent's hydrological apex at Glacier's Triple Divide Peak, water flows to three oceans: westward into tributaries of the Flathead River and then the Columbia River and the Pacific Ocean; northward into streamlets of the Saint Mary River, Oldman River, and Saskatchewan River to Nelson River and finally the Hudson Bay; and eastward into frothing Atlantic Creek to Cutback Creek and Marias River, then the mighty Mississippi River and drifting to the Gulf of Mexico.

Glacier became America's 10th national park in 1910, thanks to the Blackfeet Indian Nation selling much of the Land of the Shining Mountains to the U.S. government for establishing the park. While Glacier's nearly two dozen glaciers dominate visitors' discussions, the park was named for the glacier-carved topography, which is easily recognized by the U-shaped valleys carved by glaciers during the last ice age some 10,000 years ago. Today, Glacier visitors follow more than 740 miles of established trails.

Waterton Lakes was established initially as Kootenay Lakes Forest Park in 1895. It was renamed Waterton Lakes National Park soon after, becoming Canada's fourth national park. The park, dominated by its namesake—the 7-mile-long, 0.5-mile-wide, 487-foot-deep Upper Waterton Lake—is named for a prominent British naturalist, Sir Charles Waterton, who never visited the area but instead was honored with the naming by Lieutenant Thomas Blakiston, a member of the Palliser Expedition. Blakiston probably was the first European to visit Waterton Lakes in 1858. Interestingly enough, Waterton is the site of Canada's first oil-producing well in the West, with the 1901 Discovery Well pumping 300 barrels per day near today's Akamina Parkway, about 5 miles from the townsite of Waterton. Today, visitors enjoy 120 miles of trails.

UNESCO named the two parks the world's first International Peace Park in 1932 and a World Heritage site in 1995 for the distinctive climate, geography, hydrographic divide, and diverse flora and fauna. Additionally, UNESCO named both parks Biosphere Reserves because of the innovative approaches to sustaining a balance of biological diversity, economic development, and cultural values. Together, the parks cover 1,802 square miles.

Geography, Topography, and Geology

The Continental Divide forms the backbone of both parks, so most trails involve elevation changes and, in some cases, dramatic climbs and descents. The two parks offer a stratigraphic record of some 1,250 million years, as revealed in sedimentary rock and tectonic progression. The topography's story is told in the exposed rock, Precambrian Belt Series sedimentary rock dating back 1,600 to 800 million years. Uplift occurred 65 million to 70 million years ago, when the Belt Series pushed older Belt rock east and over the top of a younger Cretaceous formation, the Lewis Overthrust. Hikers can find ancient fossils of blue-green algae called stromatolites, Proterozoic life from the Belt Sea. Visitors will also find colorful argillite and quartzite on mountainsides and around the trails of what was once compressed under the inland seawater.

Most notably, of course, are Glacier and Waterton's deep glaciated valleys crafted by dynamic glaciers as they melted and refroze, most recently during the last ice age, which ended about 10,000 years ago. At that time, ice was a mile deep in some areas. The results are dramatic. For example, the Garden Wall, which is above Going-to-the-Sun Road, is a sawtooth arête, a knife-edged section of the Continental Divide, formed by two glaciers, one on either side of the divide. Other interesting geologic formations, such as natural amphitheater-shaped mountain cirques, also sculpted by glaciers, are visible as well. Glacial tarns are the high alpine lakes in the cirques. Sometimes, a

Research in the National Parks

Glacier National Park fosters several research projects regarding climate change, fire ecology, natural resources, and cultural resources. Perhaps the study with the most media attention is the grizzly bear research conducted by the park's Crown of the Continent Research Learning Center (CCRLC); the national forest; Montana Fish, Wildlife & Parks; the U.S. Geological Survey; and the U.S. Fish & Wildlife Service. The bear hair DNA study began in 1988 to determine the number of bears and their distribution throughout the 8-million-acre Northern Continental Divide region. Findings from 34,000 hair samples determined that 765 grizzly bears live in the region, and most are concentrated in and around Glacier. Hikers may find strands of barbed wire attached to trees to capture bear hair. Other research projects, such as monitoring the melting glaciers, may have markers in the snow or on rocks. Researchers may be in the field and available to answer questions, but they request that the public refrain from touching research sites.

Visitors can engage in the Citizen Science program at Glacier National Park. The CCRLC coordinates events, which are listed at **crownscience.org.** Many events are free and open to the public. Current Citizen Science research studies include field surveys on common loons, High Country surveys to collect data on mountain goats and pikas, and documenting five noxious weeds along Glacier's 743 miles of established trails. Glacier hosts brown bag presentations from researchers April–October in the Glacier National Park Community Building.

The annual Science & History Day is an invitation to the public to join park scientists in the Falls Theatre in Waterton Lakes National Park, usually in late July, for a free day of events and lectures.

series of tarns occur, each lower in elevation than the previous one; these are called paternoster lakes because they resemble rosary beads.

First Peoples

Evidence suggests that early explorers used the Glacier and Waterton area at least 10,000 years ago. Little is known about the early visitors, but by the late 1780s, the Southern Piikani, a branch of the Blackfeet Indians (or *Niitsitapi*), dominated the plains, hunted bison, and traveled into what is today the national park. On the west side of the mountains, the Kootenai, Salish, and Kalispel [sic] Indians fished and camped, most notably catching whitefish and drying them to store for winter sustenance. The Northern Piikani, the Blood Indians, controlled lands of Waterton and east onto the Canadian plains. The Museum of the Plains Indians in Browning, Montana, offers a well-told glimpse of Blackfeet heritage. Additionally, Sun Tours provides interpretive van tours within the parks, revealing Glacier's importance to the Blackfeet Indian Nation and focusing on history, culture, and the landscape the Indians called the Backbone of the World. Currently, the Blackfeet Nation encompasses 3,000 square miles and shares Glacier's eastern boundary with 7,000 enrolled members living on reservation lands. The Blackfeet Nation is one of seven Indian nations in Montana. The Blood Indian Reserve in Alberta, Canada, is 545 square miles, the largest in Canada, and has a population of fewer than 5,000 members living on tribal lands.

Flora

Five different ecoregions exist within Glacier and Waterton Lakes National Parks, including the alpine tundra, subalpine forest, montane forest, aspen parkland, and fescue grasslands. At least 1,132 species of vascular plants flourish in the parks, including 20 tree species, 93 shrubs and vines, 88 annuals or biennials, and 804 herbs. Researchers identify 127 nonnative plant species. Moss and lichens make up 855 nonvascular plants, joined by more than 200 fungi species. Remarkably, 30 endemic species—plants that only occur in the Northern Rocky Mountains—reside in the park.

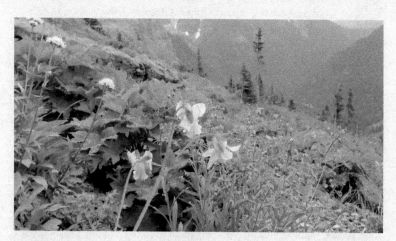

Columbine blooms *nearly everywhere in Glacier and Waterton Lakes National Parks, including here along the Boulder Pass Trail.*

Showy and memorable is beargrass, 4-foot-tall stalky plants with a mass of tiny white blossoms that grow in a clump and resemble a lantern. Each beargrass plant blooms every five to seven years, and, in some summers, hillsides seem to explode with them. Fragrant huckleberry, a deciduous shrub, grows in the moist understory of the montane and subalpine regions, often near beargrass. Sweet, purple huckleberries ripen in July and August, attracting bears and other animals. Also fragrant are the western red cedar trees, ancient and huge, shading trails near Lake McDonald. The Trail of the Cedars offers a close-up view of the 500-year-old trees growing in their easternmost habitat.

Please take heed: While eating a few berries is fine, harvesting huckleberries or other plants for use as food or medicine is prohibited in the park. Don't pick the flowers—instead, leave them for others to enjoy. Glacier National Park maintains a native plant nursery to annually supply about 50 revegetation projects.

Fauna

Nearly all of the mammal species that occurred in Glacier and Waterton National Parks prior to park designation still exist, the exceptions being bison and woodland caribou. The bison's demise occurred in the 1800s, when humans slaughtered nearly 50 million of them for meat, hides, and recreational hunting. However, small bison herds reside outside Glacier on the Blackfeet Reservation and near Waterton's boundary. Caribou, a critically endangered mammal, is now found only in extreme Northern Idaho and very occasionally Northwest Montana.

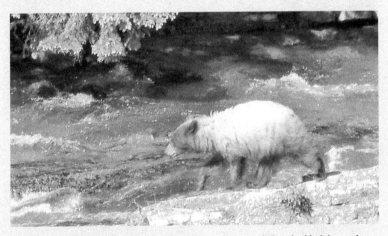

Researchers estimate *that 600 black bears roam Glacier, including this black bear cub on the Otokomi Lake Trail.*

Bear Safety

Some trails may be posted closed due to bear activity. Bears are generally more active predawn, in the evening hours, and at night. No matter where and when you hike, always take the following precautions:

- Check at entrance stations or visitor centers for bear activity or trail closures.
- Watch the bear safety video online or at park visitor centers.
- Hike in groups of three or more, make noise, and stay on the established trail.
- Carry bear-deterrent spray in an easy-to-access place, such as a holster, and know how to use it.
- Watch for signs of bears, from footprints and scat to the smell of carcasses, which attract the ursine.
- Do not pack strong-smelling food, which may draw bears' attention, and if picnicking, do not leave food or packs unattended.
- Do not run on the park trails because joggers tend to surprise bears, which in turn may instinctively chase the runner.
- Follow park guidelines for camping, food storage, and food hanging.
- Report any interactions with bears to the rangers.

If you do encounter a bear, the National Park Service suggests:

- Stay calm. Do not run. Do not make sudden movements.
- Back away slowly. Do not drop your backpack—keep it on your back in case you need it for protection.
- Speak quietly to the bear but don't shout.
- Avoid looking directly at the bear, as biologists believe that the bear may sense a challenge. Instead, turn sideways and assume a nonthreatening posture.
- If a bear does charge, try not to run, and instead fall on the ground protecting your chest, stomach, and head. Often, bears will make a bluff charge, veer off into the woods, and be gone.

Most visitors will see the flashy white mountain goats on Logan Pass at the summit of Going-to-the-Sun Road and on surrounding cliffs as the even-toed ungulate scrambles over rocks, nibbling lichen, herbs, moss, and grass. While the billy goats, nanny goats, and kids may approach visitors and seem curious, it is illegal to approach or touch any wild animal in the parks. Instead, photographs of Glacier and Waterton's 66 native mammal species will provide lasting memories. Large carnivores, such as grizzly bears, black bears, gray wolves, mountain lions, wolverines, and Canada lynx, thrive here. Grizzly bears and Canada lynx are federally listed threatened species, while the gray wolf, bald eagle, and peregrine falcon were once threatened and endangered species that have recovered and have been delisted.

Researchers estimate that about 300 grizzly bears and 600 black bears roam Glacier National Park, with a few dozen each within Waterton Lakes National Park. Since 1988, researchers have been conducting a DNA hair study and using remote camera systems to document the ursine residents. For more on this study, see the sidebar on page 3.

Other large mammals that visitors encounter are elk, deer, and moose. Elk most likely will be found on the prairies on the east side of both Glacier and Waterton National Parks, although the 500-pound elk cows and 700-pound bulls do cruise the timber on both sides of the Continental Divide. Only male elk have antlers, which are shed each spring and regrown summer though fall.

Mule and white-tailed deer live in all but the rockiest, snowiest elevations of Glacier and Waterton. Mule deer, sometimes called black-tailed deer, are found in open forests, meadows, and the higher alpine regions of the parks. White-tailed deer are distinguished from mule deer by their smaller ears and distinctive white tail. White-tailed deer tend to reside in coniferous forests, meadows, creeks, and river bottoms. Only the bucks grow antlers, which are shed each spring and regrown summer through fall.

Moose thrive in the parks' coniferous forests, but most are seen by visitors as the moose search for food in lakes, streams, and marshy areas, where they eat willows, sedges, and marsh grasses. Moose are exceedingly large and unpredictable vegetarians. Some bull elk reach nearly 7 feet tall and 1,000 pounds. Moose are the second-largest land mammal in North America, behind the bison, and the largest member of the deer family. The quadrupeds live mostly solitary lives, except during breeding season and when cows have calves. Only the bulls grow the large palmate antlers, which they shed annually. Bulls also sport a thicket of skin and hair called a dewlap that dangles under the moose's chin.

Another large mammal, the bighorn sheep, nibbles grasses, sedges, and lichens on both sides of the Continental Divide. The bighorns, recognizable by the large, curled horns on the rams and the thin, straighter horns on the ewes, live year-round in the alpine zone. The light-brown to grayish fur on most of the body provides good camouflage. Their white rumps and back legs are often what catch the hiker's eye. Bighorn sheep tend to gather in flocks of ewes, lambs, and rams. During mating season, the fall rut, the rams battle for dominance and breeding rights by running full tilt at each other and crashing skulls together. The clashes are fascinating to watch—and hear. The skull-cracking sounds echo from the mountainsides. Thanks to adaptations, such as enlarged corneal and frontal sinuses and bony septa, the male bighorn rarely

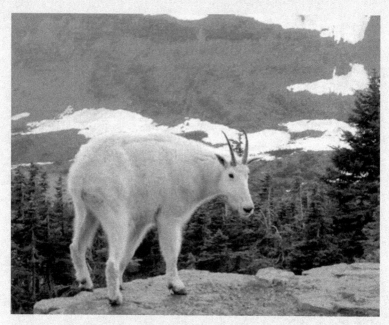

The iconic mountain goat *is Glacier's native goodwill ambassador, often posing for photos at the Hidden Lake Overlook above Logan Pass.*

sustain brain injuries during the impact. The bighorn sheep is the provincial mammal of Alberta.

Other wildlife that visitors will likely encounter include coyotes, river otters, mink, marten, and weasels. Visitors often hear pikas and marmots, chipmunks, and the golden-mantled ground squirrel. Evenings, you may see the little brown bat, long-legged bat, big brown bat, and silver-haired bat. A few rare creatures include the northern bog lemming, native to coniferous forests; the Richardson ground squirrel and the thirteen-lined ground squirrel, both grasslands residents; porcupines; jackrabbits; cottontail rabbits; red foxes; bobcats; long-eared bats; hoary bats; and the fisher. The parks' ranger-led evening programs sometimes detail the various mammals. Some of the lodges, especially Lake McDonald Lodge, have mounted wildlife on display. A mammal checklist is available online and at park entrance stations.

Numerous birds flock to Glacier and Waterton, thanks to the terrestrial, aquatic, and riparian habitats. Golden eagles cruise the Crown of the Continent each spring and fall, using the thermals to glide between nesting areas in Canada and Alaska and winter homes in the southern United States and Mexico. Bald eagles can be found nearly year-round in the parks. Occasionally, portions of some lakes are closed to visitors during the eagle-nesting season. Glacier is a good place to watch the rare harlequin ducks—visitors may encounter researchers as they document the "clown ducks" in McDonald Creek, where the birds search for mollusks and aquatic insects. Most often, visitors will see Canada geese, mallard ducks, and dippers, or water ouzels, in and near the lakes. The parks' websites have bird checklists that list the 260 species of birds that reside here at least some of the year.

When to Go

Both Glacier and Waterton Lakes National Parks are open year-round; however, snow-covered access roads prevent most people from visiting during the long winter. Most visitors see the parks' glistening peaks, spectacular waterfalls, aquamarine lakes, and dashing wildlife between June and October. Depending on how much snow accumulates from November to May, some high-elevation trails may remain snow-covered well into July. Going-to-the-Sun Road, in general, opens in June after snowplows cut through deep avalanche debris and drifts. The historic road closes in late October or early November, depending on snow. An 8-mile section of the road from West Glacier to Lake McDonald Lodge remains open year-round. July and August see the bulk of visitors to both parks; hotels and park campgrounds tend to be full for a few weeks in late July, although several lodgings and campgrounds may have openings just outside park boundaries.

Weather and Seasons

Since snow may fall any month of the year, visitors are advised to bring a variety of clothing and wear layers, including wicking material closest to skin, a thermal wool or synthetic sweater, and wind- and weatherproof outer layers—both top and bottom. Always pack a warm hat and gloves; a brilliant sunrise might suggest a warm day, but Mother Nature makes fools of those who don't pack extra clothing. The parks have registered 80-degree temperature swings within a few hours, often preceded by high winds. In general, May and June are known for mixed days of sun, rain, or snow, while July through early October are dry with cool to cold nights. Cross-country skiing and snowshoeing on trails and closed roads are common November through March and in some places even into May.

Spring comes late to the Northern Rockies. Spring hikes, mid- to late May, begin and venture through lower elevations or climb south-facing slopes where the sun melts the snow earlier than in other locales. For example, in the West Glacier area, much of the trail to the Apgar Lookout will be snow-free by late May, although the trail is likely to remain muddy for another month. Spring hikes are rewarding, in that few people are out on the trails and visitors may see more wildlife, especially birds. Bears emerge from their dens in spring, with the male bears, the boars, emerging earlier than sows with cubs. Bears can often be spotted this time of year digging through avalanche debris as they look for carrion, mostly mountain goats, that perished in avalanches. Note that many lodging properties and campgrounds do not open until June.

Summers generally offer moderate to warm temperatures. Because the trails reach high elevations and sometimes cross or amble near snowfields, travelers should be prepared with sunscreen, sturdy hiking boots, and a hiking pole. If crossing a snowfield, be aware that savvy hikers use crampons, hiking poles, or ski poles for safety. If it's exceedingly icy, however, it's best to find an alternate route around the snow or access that trail later in the year. The park service trail crew posts trail conditions with updates added often (**nps.gov/glac/planyourvisit/trailstatusreports.htm**). Park service rangers lead hikes during the summer; the ranger-led hikes are posted in the park's free newspaper.

Fall is often the local hikers' favorite time to visit Glacier and Waterton Lakes because the aspens shimmer gold, the daytime temperatures allow for cool to warm hiking, and few other humans venture into the backcountry. Fall is also when hikers may hear bugling, the bull elk's call to females and his warning to other bulls. And most importantly, fall is when grizzly and black bears prepare for hibernation, which includes eating mass quantities of food, a stage called hyperphagia. The bears eat nearly constantly to add weight before heading to dens, usually after the first snows.

Winter is the silent season in Glacier and Waterton, yet it is very much a lively and active time in the parks. Skiers and snowshoers can join guides to access special and spectacular places, tailored to the visitors' fitness and abilities. In Glacier, the Apgar Ranger Station opens daily for limited visitor services. Waterton's offices are closed for most public services, and the Waterton Township has few open facilities and businesses in winter, although several cross-country ski trails lead from the community and into the backcountry. Designated winter trails are groomed for weekend cross-country skiing,

Average High and Low Temperature (°F) by Month, West Glacier						
	JAN	**FEB**	**MAR**	**APR**	**MAY**	**JUNE**
High	31°	35°	43°	54°	65°	72°
Low	18°	19°	25°	31°	38°	44°
	JULY	**AUG**	**SEPT**	**OCT**	**NOV**	**DEC**
High	80°	79°	68°	52°	37°	29°
Low	49°	47°	39°	32°	26°	18°

including the Cameron Ski Trail and the Dipper Ski Trail. Skiers should check in with the Waterton Warden's Office for voluntary self-registration both before and upon returning from winter trips. Winter ski maps are available both on the parks' websites and at the Apgar Ranger Station. Ski touring groups departing from established winter trails should pack avalanche transceiver beacons and shovels, have knowledge of avalanche conditions and self-rescue responsibilities, and have checked with the local warden in Waterton at 403-859-2224 or the Canadian Avalanche Association at 800-667-1105. The Flathead Avalanche Center's forecast for Glacier is available at **flathead avalanche.org** or the advisory hot line at 406-257-8402.

Fees, Camping, and Permits

Backcountry Permit applications are available online at **nps.gov/glac/plan yourvisit/backcountry.htm,** and for walk-ins at the Apgar Backcountry Permit Office, open May 1 through late September, daily, 7 a.m.–4:30 p.m. and late September to October 31, daily, 8 a.m.–3:30 p.m. The Apgar Backcountry Permit Office is closed November through April. Note that **Glacier Guides** (406-387-5555; **glacierguides.com**) offers guided trips into the backcountry from one night to two weeks.

Biking and Boating

Glacier National Park Bicycling and Spring Bicycling Season (when roads are closed to motor vehicles)

Because few roads crisscross Glacier, the main roads tend to carry significant traffic from June to Labor Day; therefore, the park restricts cyclists to certain times of day on the Going-to-the-Sun Road, when fewer motor vehicles converge on the historic route. Cyclists are prohibited on Going-to-the-Sun Road from Apgar Campground to Sprague Creek Campground and also from Logan Creek to Logan Pass eastbound (the uphill portion on the west side of Logan Pass) between 11 a.m. and 4 p.m. Cyclists tackling the 50-mile road and the 3,477-foot climb from Apgar over Logan Pass should start early in the day, recognize that there is no available water or food after Lake McDonald Lodge, and plan on 45 minutes of pedaling from Sprague Creek to Logan Creek and 3 hours of riding from Logan Creek to Logan Pass.

During spring, a portion of Going-to-the Sun Road is open to foot and bike traffic after snow is gone from the lower elevations and while snow removal continues above the Loop on the West Side and above Siyeh Bend on the East Side. Check locally because snow depths vary from year to year.

Family-Friendly Overnight Backpacking

For an introduction to backpacking, families will find excellent views, gentle trails, and quiet campsites at numerous locations. On the West Side of the Continental Divide in the North Fork, the 5.5-mile Logging Lake Trail is a good introduction to backpacking, thanks to gentle gain in elevation, outstanding views, and a rewarding lake swim. Backpackers might extend the stay with an additional 2.6 miles to Adair Campground, also on Logging Lake, or even to Grace Lake, another 4.6 miles from the Logging Lake Campground.

In the Two Medicine area, Cobalt Lake offers a thrilling backcountry experience, where even in July, snow will cling to shady spots. The hike, inclusive of the boat shuttle, is 4.4 miles each way.

From Waterton, one of the more unique backcountry camping experiences includes a boat ride across Upper Waterton Lake to Goat Haunt (passports are required), and the easy 0.25-mile hike to the Goat Haunt Shelters. These three-sided, wooden shelters have concrete floors and roofs and allow backpackers space and shelter to set up tents inside while cooking in a common area. Many day hikes depart from Goat Haunt. Reservations are necessary through the Apgar Backcountry Permit Office.

Due to continued road construction, sections of Going-to-the Sun Road (and often other park roads) may lack pavement and may be covered with jagged rock, mud, and snow. The road may have entire sections closed for construction, may be closed overnight for construction, and closes each fall through late spring due to snow. Construction delays may last up to 30 minutes. Check with the rangers for dates and details at **nps.gov/glac** or 406-888-7800.

Bicycles are not allowed in Glacier's backcountry. Bicycles are allowed in campgrounds on the paved and gravel roads and the Apgar Bike Trail, 2.6 miles to West Glacier. Additionally, cyclists enjoy the 5-mile ride from West Glacier (on the access road to the Apgar Lookout Trailhead) on the Old Flathead Ranger Station route, along a former jeep trail that follows the Middle Fork of the Flathead River. Many cyclists discover the 28-mile gravel Inside North Fork Road from Fish Creek Campground to Polebridge, which is mostly free of motor vehicles; however, in spring and early summer, downed trees may impede travel. Washouts at stream crossings and often a big washout at Logging Creek Campground make portions of the road impassable—check with the rangers regarding road conditions. Note that bears and other wild animals frequent the roads and trails; it's best to bike in groups, carry bear spray, and make lots of noise.

Bicycle rentals are available in Whitefish at **Glacier Cyclery** (**glacier cyclery.com** or 406-862-6446), **Great Northern Cycles** (**greatnorthern cycles.com** or 406-862-6446), and **Paddlefish Sports** (**paddlefish-sports .com** or 406-260-7733).

Waterton Backcountry Biking

Waterton National Park allows bicycles on five designated backcountry and frontcountry trails. Akamina Pass Trail begins on Akamina Parkway and climbs to the Continental Divide and the boundary of Waterton and Akamina-Kishinena Provincial Park, then on to Wall Lake for a 10.4-kilometer/6.4-mile round-trip. Crandell Mountain Loop is accessible from three trailheads for the challenging 20.6-kilometer/12.8-mile ride on steep, rocky, and washout terrain. The loop includes riding on portions of Akamina Parkway and Waterton Townsite streets. The 6.9-kilometer/4.25-mile Kootenai Brown Trail is a gentle, paved multiuse route through Townsite Campground and the community to the visitor facility and the Waterton Valley (motorized vehicles are prohibited). The 13.2-kilometer/8.2-mile one-way Snowshoe Trail begins at the Red Rock Canyon parking lot and is popular with beginner bicyclists. The 10.5-kilometer/6.5-mile Wishbone Trail begins on the Chief Mountain Highway, 0.5 kilometer south of the junction with Highway 5, and challenges cyclists to a ford crossing of Sofa Creek en route to the Wishbone dock on Middle Waterton Lake. Bicycle rentals are available in Waterton Townsite at **Pat's Gas & Cycle Rental** (403-859-2266). Cyclists should be aware that hikers, horseback riders, and wildlife may be on the trails. Overnight bicycle trips require a wilderness use permit, available at 403-859-5133 or **pc.gc.ca.**

Boat Rentals

Most park rivers are not navigable for canoeing, kayaking, or rafting; however, lake boat rentals are available at Apgar, Lake McDonald, Two Medicine Lake, Many Glacier, and Saint Mary Lake. Glacier Park Boat Company's rates and season are posted at **glacierparkboats.com,** or call 406-257-2426 for more information.

In Waterton Lakes National Park, boat rentals are available at Cameron Lake Boat Rentals; visit **cameronlakeboatrentals.com** or call 403-859-2396 for more information.

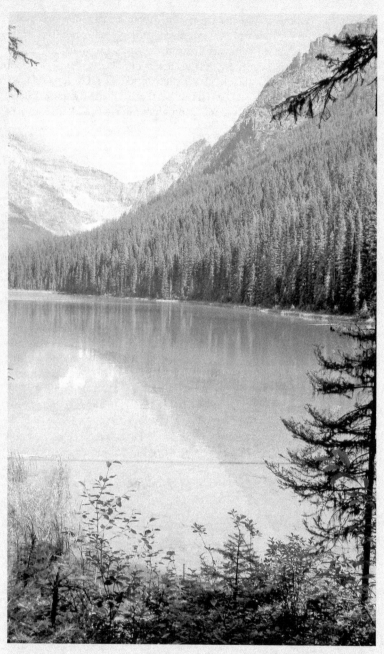

Akokala Lake; *see profile 11, page 83.*

On the Trail

Every outing should begin with proper preparation, which usually takes only a few minutes. Even the easiest trail can turn up unexpected surprises. People seldom think about getting lost or injured, but unexpected things can and do happen. Simple precautions can make the difference between a good story and a dangerous situation.

Use the Top Trails ratings and descriptions to determine whether a particular trail is a good match with your fitness and energy level, given current conditions and time of year. Always hike with companions. Always carry bear-deterrent spray, and know how to use it. Heed trail closures posted at trailheads or trail junctions—rangers may close trails to keep nesting eagles at peace, to keep hikers from stumbling upon aggressive bears or other wildlife, or to prevent visitors from accessing trails with unstable footing.

Have a Plan

Choose wisely The first step to enjoying any trail is to match the trail to your abilities. It's no use overestimating your experience or fitness; know your abilities and limitations, and use the Top Trails difficulty rating that accompanies each trail.

Leave word about your plans The most basic of precautions is leaving word of your intentions with friends or family. Each of the park hotels offers guests a free sign-in sheet to leave with the front desk, stating day, time and place of hike, and expected return time. Many people will hike the backcountry their entire lives without ever relying on this safety net, but establishing this simple habit is free insurance.

Bathers Beware

More people die in Glacier National Park each year in water accidents than for any other reason. The snow and glacial melt-water career down mountainsides in unpredictable surges, yet the water rarely warms enough for sustained swimming. Lake temperatures rarely warm above 45–55°F, creating the potential for hypothermia.

Prepare and Plan

- Know your abilities and limitations.
- Leave word about your plans.
- Know the area and the route.

It's best to leave specific information—location, trail name, intended time of travel—with a responsible person. However, if this is not possible or if plans change at the last minute, you should still check in at a ranger station, trail register, or visitor center if there is one.

Review the route Before embarking on any hike, read the entire description, and study the map. It isn't necessary to memorize every detail, but it is worthwhile to have a clear mental picture of the trail and the general area.

If the trail or terrain has complex intersections, augment the trail guide with a topographic map. Maps and current weather and trail-condition information are often available at local ranger and park stations, hotel gift shops, and local stores, and these resources should be used.

Carry the Essentials

Proper preparation for any type of trail includes gathering essential items. Trip checklists will vary tremendously by trail and conditions.

Clothing When the weather is good, light, comfortable clothing is the obvious choice. It's easy to believe that very little spare clothing is needed, but a prepared hiker has something tucked away for any emergency, from a surprise snow shower to an unexpected overnight stay in a remote area.

Clothing includes proper footwear, essential for hiking the trails. As a trail becomes more demanding, you will need footwear that performs. Running shoes are fine for many trails. If you will be carrying substantial weight or encountering sustained rugged terrain, step up to hiking boots.

In hot, sunny weather, proper clothing includes a hat, sunglasses, a long-sleeved shirt, and sunscreen. In cooler weather, particularly when it's wet, carry waterproof outerwear and quick-drying undergarments (avoid cotton). As a general rule, whatever the conditions, bring layers that can be combined or removed to provide comfort and protection from the elements in a wide variety of conditions.

Water Never embark on a trail without carrying water. At all times, particularly in warm weather, adequate water is of key importance. Experts recommend at least 2 quarts of water per person per day. When hiking in

Trail Essentials

- Dress to keep cool, but be ready for cold.
- Bring plenty of water and adequate food.

heat, a gallon or more may be appropriate. At the extreme, dehydration can be life threatening. More commonly, inadequate water brings fatigue and muscle aches.

For most outings, unless the day is very hot or the trail very long, you should plan to carry sufficient water for the entire trail. Unfortunately, in North America, natural water sources are questionable, generally loaded with various risks, including bacteria, viruses, and fertilizers. The snow may also have bacteria that can make you ill.

Water treatment If it's necessary to make use of trailside water, you should filter or treat it. There are three methods for treating water: boiling, chemical treatment, and filtering. Boiling is best but often impractical, as it requires a heat source, a pot, and time. Chemical treatments, available in sporting goods stores, handle some problems, including the troublesome giardia parasite, but will not combat many man-made chemical pollutants. The preferred method is filtration, which removes giardia and other contaminants and doesn't leave any unpleasant aftertaste.

If this hasn't convinced you to carry all the water you need, here's one final admonishment: Be prepared for surprises. Water sources described in the text or on maps may be frozen over, change course, or dry up completely. Never run your water bottle dry in expectation of the next source; fill up and filter when water is available, and always keep a little in reserve.

Food While not as critical as water, food is energy, and its importance shouldn't be underestimated. Avoid foods that are hard to digest, such as candy bars and potato chips. Carry high energy, fast-digesting foods, such as nutrition bars, dried fruit, gorp, and jerky. Bring a little extra food—it's good protection against an outing that turns unexpectedly long, perhaps due to weather or losing your way.

Useful but Less than Essential Items

Navigation devices (and the know-how to use them) Many trails don't require much navigation—meaning a map and compass or GPS device aren't always as essential as water or food—but it can be a close call. If the trail is remote or infrequently visited, consider a contour map and compass to be necessities.

A handheld GPS is a useful trail companion, but it's no substitute for a map and compass; knowing your longitude and latitude is not much help without a map. On some trail sections, GPS units won't work due to the mountains or canyon walls.

Cell phone Most parts of the country, even remote destinations, have some level of cellular coverage. In extreme circumstances, a cell phone can be a lifesaver. But don't depend on it in mountainous terrain; coverage is unpredictable and batteries fail. And be sure that the occasion warrants the phone call—a blister doesn't justify a call to search and rescue.

Gear Depending on the remoteness and rigor of the trail, there are many additional useful items to consider: pocketknife, flashlight, fire source (waterproof matches, lighter, or flint), emergency shelter blanket, and first-aid kit.

Every member of your party should carry the appropriate essential items described above, as well as a canister of bear-deterrent spray since groups often split up or get separated and spread out along the trail. Solo hikers should be even more disciplined about preparation and carry more gear. Traveling solo is inherently more risky, especially in grizzly bear country. Solo travel is discouraged—instead, join a ranger-led hike or hire a guide.

Trail Etiquette

The overriding rule on the trail is "Leave No Trace." Interest in visiting natural areas continues to increase in North America, even as the quantity of unspoiled natural areas continues to shrink. These pressures make it ever more critical that we leave no trace of our visits.

Never litter If you carried it in, it's easy enough to carry it out. Leave the trail in the same, if not better, condition than you find it. Try picking up any litter you encounter and packing it out—it's a great feeling. Just one piece of garbage, and you've made a difference.

Stay on the trail Paths have been created, sometimes over many years, for many purposes: to protect the surrounding natural areas, to avoid dangers, and to provide the best route. Leaving the trail can cause damage that takes

 Trail Etiquette

- Leave no trace. Never litter.
- Stay on the trail. Never cut switchbacks.
- Share the trail. Use courtesy and common sense.
- Leave it there.
- Don't disturb wildlife.

years to undo. Never cut switchbacks. Shortcutting rarely saves energy or time, and it takes a terrible toll on the land, trampling precious native plant life and hastening erosion. Moreover, safety and consideration intersect on the trail. It's hard to get truly lost if you stay on the trail.

Share the trail The best trails attract many visitors, and you should be prepared to share the trail with others. Do your part to minimize impact.

Commonly accepted trail etiquette dictates that cyclists yield to both hikers and equestrians, hikers yield to horseback riders, downhill hikers yield to uphill hikers, and everyone stays to the right. Not everyone knows these rules of the road, so let common sense and good humor be the final guide.

Leave it there Destruction or removal of plants and animals, or historical, prehistoric, or geological items, is certainly unethical and almost always illegal.

Getting lost If you become lost, stay on the trail. Stop and take stock of the situation. In many cases, a few minutes of calm reflection will yield a solution. Consider all the clues available; use the sun to identify directions if you don't have a compass. If you determine that you are indeed lost, stay on the main trail, and stay put. You are more likely to encounter other people if you stay in one place.

A Note from the Author/Photographer

I am lucky. I've been hiking, biking, paddling, and skiing through Glacier National Park and Waterton Lakes National Park since the 1970s, and I have met many good friends on these trails. When our children were too small for their own hiking boots, my husband and I placed them in canoes or in child carrier backpacks and discovered the parks' wonders through their eyes. Now, as college students, they enjoy the parks at their speed. I'd like to thank my husband, Lynn Sellegren, and kids, Gretchen and Bridger Sellegren, for joining me on most of the two parks' 860 miles of trails. We also had lots of fun trail days and camping nights with my in-laws, Mona Sellegren and Chuck Kempner, who hiked with the Over The Hill Gang of mostly retirees, another group deserving a tip of the hat for their decades-long participation as volunteers in Glacier. My gratitude also extends to all my ski-booted and hiking friends who joined me in the past few years while I re-hiked the trails detailed in this book. They include Laura Strong, Nancy Persons, Wendy Pierce, Linda and Carl Pittman, Cyndy Braun, and Nancy Braun. A note of gratitude also goes to Montana's Office of Tourism, Glacier Park Boat Company, Glacier Gateway Outfitters, Mystery Ranch Backpacks, Glacier Park, Inc., Izaak Walton Inn, Glacier National Park, Waterton Lakes National Park, and Garmin.

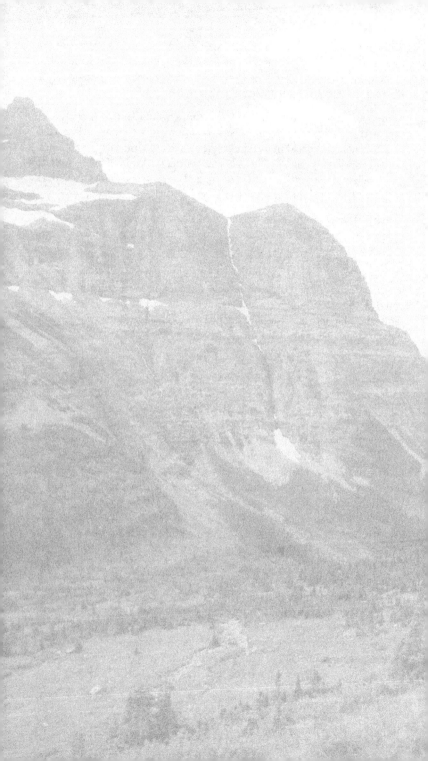

CHAPTER 1

West Side Trails: Lake McDonald Area and the North Fork

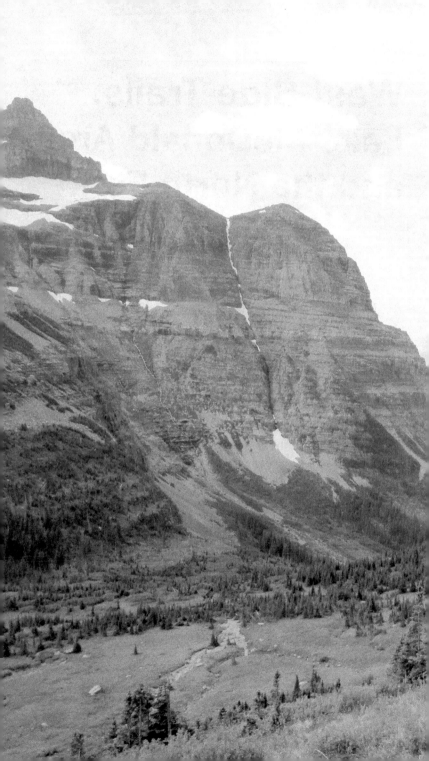

West Side Trails: Lake McDonald Area and the North Fork

Glacier National Park's western half is dominated by lush forests, emerald and turquoise lakes, and the Pacific Maritime climate impacting an ecosystem that hangs under the Continental Divide's western shoulder. It's here that temperate, wet Pacific Northwest meteorological conditions sustain the northern alpine forests, wetlands, and riparian areas. The West Glacier park entrance welcomes visitors year-round, although the community of West Glacier seems to hibernate much of the winter—a few eateries and lodging facilities remain open. Apgar Campground remains open year-round but has limited services in winter. In Apgar, visitors will also find the Apgar Ranger Station and Apgar Backcountry Office, as well as restaurants, gift shops, a motel, cabins, boat rentals, and scenery beyond compare. Lake McDonald dominates the view to the north, hugged by forested slopes and snowcapped peaks. At the horizon, the Continental Divide lines the background like a picket fence, and indeed, it's called the Garden Wall. Lake McDonald Lodge perches on the southeast shore near Sprague Creek Campground. While Lake McDonald is among the park's largest lochs at 9.9 by 5.2 miles, a series of big lakes punctuates the glaciated valleys of the West Side. Many lakes are only accessible via trail; however, the rough North Fork Road leads to the tiny town of Polebridge, Montana, and the Polebridge Ranger Station entrance gate. Single-lane gravel roads crawl to the lovely Bowman and Kintla Lakes and lakeside campgrounds. Polebridge itself is known for the fresh-baked pastries made daily at the century-old Polebridge Mercantile, the live music on the lawn of the Northern Lights Saloon, its outdoor volleyball court, and fantastic stargazing (the town lacks electricity). The two dozen full-time residents rely on solar energy, tiny

Opposite and overleaf: *From the Boulder Pass Trail above Brown Pass, the view down to Bowman Lake sparkles with wildflowers and the shimmering Thunderbird Glacier.*

23

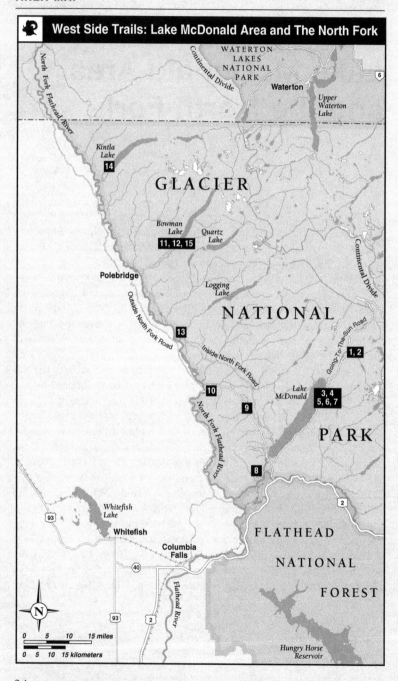

West Side Trails: Lake McDonald Area and The North Fork

West Side Trails: Lake McDonald Area and the North Fork

TRAIL	DIFFICULTY	LENGTH	TYPE	USES & ACCESS	TERRAIN	FLORA & FAUNA	OTHER
1	1	0.95	Loop	Day Hiking, Child-Friendly, Wheelchair Access		Flora, Birds, Wildlife	Secluded, Views
2	2	5.8	Out-and-back	Day Hiking, Child-Friendly	Lake	Flora, Wildlife	Geologic Interest
3	4	12.4	Out-and-back	Day Hiking, Backpacking, Horses		Flora, Wildlife	Secluded, Historic Interest
4	3	8.4	Out-and-back	Day Hiking, Horses, Child-Friendly	Lake	Flora, Wildlife	Secluded, Swimming, Fishing, Views
5	2	5.8	Out-and-back	Day Hiking, Child-Friendly	Lake	Flora, Wildlife	Secluded, Fishing, Geologic Interest, Historic Interest
6	5	10.1	Out-and-back	Day Hiking		Flora, Wildlife	Secluded, Views, Geologic Interest, Historic Interest
7	1–3	16.8	Out-and-back	Child-Friendly, Ski/Snowshoe		Wildlife	Secluded, Views, Geologic Interest, Historic Interest
8	3	7.2	Out-and-back	Day Hiking, Child-Friendly		Flora, Birds, Wildlife	Secluded, Views, Photo Opportunity, Geologic Interest, Historic Interest
9	3	12.0	Out-and-back	Day Hiking		Flora, Wildlife	Secluded, Views, Geologic Interest, Historic Interest
10	1	1.0	Loop	Day Hiking, Child-Friendly		Flora, Birds, Wildlife	Secluded, Geologic Interest, Historic Interest
11	3	11.6	Out-and-back	Day Hiking, Backpacking, Child-Friendly	Lake	Flora, Wildlife, Wildfire Ecology	Secluded, Fishing, Views, Geologic Interest, Historic Interest
12	3–4	12.9	Loop	Day Hiking, Backpacking	Lake	Flora, Birds, Wildlife, Wildfire Ecology	Secluded, Fishing, Geologic Interest, Historic Interest
13	2	11.0	Out-and-back	Day Hiking, Backpacking, Child-Friendly	Lake	Flora, Birds, Wildlife	Secluded, Geologic Interest, Historic Interest
14	5	40.0	Out-and-back	Backpacking	Lake, Waterfall	Flora, Wildlife	Secluded, Fishing, Views, Geologic Interest, Historic Interest
15	5	22.3	Point-to-point	Backpacking	Lake, Waterfall	Flora, Birds, Wildlife	Secluded, Geologic Interest, Historic Interest

Legend

USES & ACCESS
- Day Hiking
- Backpacking
- Horses
- Child-Friendly
- Ski/Snowshoe
- Wheelchair Access

TYPE
- Loop
- Balloon
- Out-and-back
- Point-to-point
- DIFFICULTY - 1 2 3 4 5 + less   more

TERRAIN
- Lake
- Waterfall
- Glacier

FLORA & FAUNA
- Flora
- Birds
- Wildlife
- Wildfire Ecology

OTHER
- Secluded
- Swimming
- Fishing
- Views
- Photo Opportunity
- Geologic Interest
- Historic Interest

water-powered generation systems, gas- or diesel-powered generators, and propane gas. The "Merc" is open daily, May 1 through the end of November.

Permits and Maps

Day hikers are not required to purchase permits; however, backcountry trekkers who plan to camp at any one of the 65 backcountry campgrounds must purchase a camping permit. Permits are available at the Apgar Backcountry Office or online, where you can download a form and fax or mail it in. Last-minute campsites are a rare find from mid-July to Labor Day, so plan ahead.

A fishing permit is not required to fish in Glacier, but a Montana fishing license is required outside the park, and a Conservation/Recreation Use Permit is required for all activities on the Blackfeet Reservation (call 406-338-7207 for information). Fishing is catch-and-release only in certain areas for cutthroat trout—check with the entrance stations for details. The daily catch-and-possession limit is five fish, with a maximum of two cutthroat trout, two burbot (ling), one northern pike, two mountain whitefish, five lake whitefish, five kokanee salmon, five grayling, five rainbow trout, and five lake trout. Some waters of the West Side are closed to fishing, including Kintla Creek between Kintla Lake and Upper Kintla Lake and all of Upper Kintla Lake, Bowman Creek above Bowman Lake, and Logging Creek between Logging Lake and Grace Lake.

The following creeks are closed to fishing for their entire length: Ole, Park, Muir, Coal, Nyack, Fish, Lee, Otatso, Boulder, and Kennedy Creeks. The North Fork of the Flathead River within 200 yards of the mouth of Big Creek is also closed to fishing.

Free park maps are available at entrance stations. Each of the park's lodging properties offers rudimentary local-area maps with details of trailhead access. Excellent maps are available for purchase at the in-park bookstores, gift shops, and grocery stores, as well as through the Glacier National Park Conservancy's bookstore in the West Glacier train depot, sporting goods shops, and general stores outside the park and online.

Opposite: *Avalanche Creek along the Trail of the Cedars froths as it scours rock in the narrow Avalanche Gorge.*

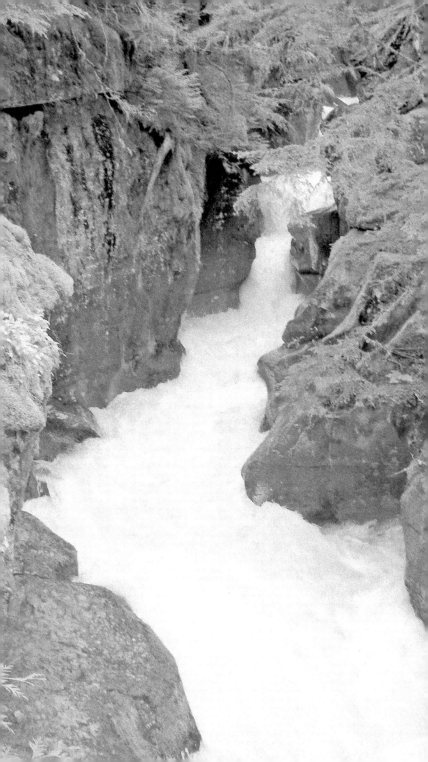

TRAIL SUMMARIES

West Side Trails: Lake McDonald Area and the North Fork

TRAIL 1

Day hiking,
child-friendly,
wheelchair accessible
0.95 mile
Loop
Difficulty 1 2 3 4 5

Trail of the Cedars.................... 33

This most popular trail in Glacier gently winds through a grove of western red cedars where the understory seldom receives much sunlight. Inviting and easy, the paved and boardwalk loop is replete with interpretive signs, benches, and a footbridge over gushing Avalanche Creek.

TRAIL 2

Day hiking,
child-friendly
5.8 miles
Out-and-back
Difficulty 1 2 3 4 5

Avalanche Lake Trail 37

A family favorite, the hike to Avalanche Lake takes about 2 hours and affords previews of several ecosystems, from the sheltered understory of 500-year-old cedar trees alongside a roiling stream to a pine forest where deer flick their tails to the final reward: emerald-green Avalanche Lake rimmed with melting snow and enlivened by mountain goats on cliffs above.

TRAIL 3

Day hiking,
backpacking, horses
12.4 miles
Out-and-back
Difficulty 1 2 3 4 5

Sperry Chalet via Gunsight Pass Trail................ 41

A challenging, 3,500-foot climb offers viewpoints at every other switchback for the first 1.5 miles. Next up is a tromp under the Douglas Fir montane, until, at last, the trees open up to reveal waterfalls, cascading streams, mountain goats, and the stunning 100-year-old Sperry Chalet, where those with reservations find elegant backcountry dining and rustic lodging, 6.2 miles from civilization.

Snyder Lake Trail 47

Families enjoy this walk, 4.4 miles each way, passing through thick timber and past huckleberry bushes to Snyder Lake. At the lake, large flat rocks provide the perfect spot for picnics below towering, snow-encrusted cliffs, where waterfalls spray down from the skirts of the Little Matterhorn and Edwards Mountain, filling the lake for the westslope cutthroat.

Fish Lake via Snyder Ridge
Fire Trail 53

A quiet lake awaits hikers who find the shady trail a lovely respite from inclement weather. This trip is a good choice in early summer, when higher-elevation routes are still cloaked in snow, keeping deer and elk at this lower elevation where pileated woodpeckers flit through the timber.

Mount Brown Lookout Trail 57

The most challenging hike in Glacier climbs 4,250 feet in 5 miles, finishing among the clouds where mountain goats roam around the lookout building. The few humans who venture here enjoy photo-worthy views of Heavens Peak, Mount Vaught, McPartland Mountain, and Sperry Glacier.

Going-to-the-Sun (Winter Trail) 63

A summer road becomes a wonderful wintry introduction to Glacier's brumal days. Cross-country skiers and snowshoers are treated to the partially frozen yet very much awake and frothy Sacred Dancing Cascade of McDonald Creek along the closed road, which is often frequented by deer and snowshoe hare.

Logging Lake Trail

As an excellent introduction to the backcountry, gentle Logging Lake Trail ambles through ponderosa pines and wildflower meadows, following Logging Creek, backdropped by mountain views now visible thanks to wildfires a decade ago.

Day hiking, backpacking, child-friendly
11.0 miles
Out-and-back
Difficulty 1 **2** 3 4 5

Boulder Pass Trail to Hole in the Wall

The backpacking trip to Hole in the Wall leads to some of the most sought-after campsites in the backcountry, but hikers must earn the mountain-cirque locale with a difficult trek, often camping partway to the head of Kintla Lake and again at Boulder Pass Campgrounds. But the rewards are many: Dozens of waterfalls, high alpine meadows, and hanging gardens decorate Hole in the Wall.

Backpacking
40.0 or 33.4 miles
Out-and-back or
point-to-point
Difficulty 1 2 3 4 **5**

Bowman Lake Trail to Goat Haunt and Waterton, Canada

This multiday backpacking trek into Glacier National Park begins among thick groves of trees, crosses the Continental Divide in the alpine ecosystem at treeline, passes sparkling lakes and shimmering waterfalls melting from glaciers, and ends at the edge of Canada's prairie grasslands of Waterton Lakes National Park.

Backpacking
22.3 miles
Point-to-point
Difficulty 1 2 3 4 **5**

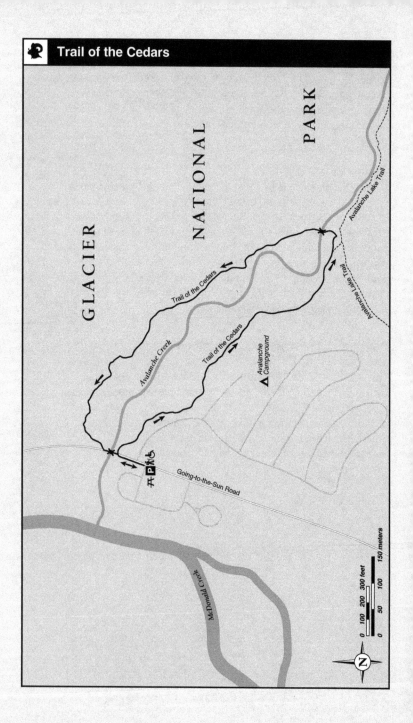

Trail of the Cedars

This loop trail circles through a grove of western red cedars, some of which are 80 feet tall and 15 feet around at the base. These lacy trees are among the easternmost groves of water-loving western red cedars—not a true cedar but an evergreen cypress and the only *Thuja* species native to western North America. Its flat and lacy foliage is fragrant when crushed. Trail of the Cedars is a must-do hike for all visitors and a fine choice for the first hike of a park visit. It exemplifies why Glacier is unique; the 1.2-million-acre park encompasses three very different ecosystems. The microclimate here is more akin to the Pacific Northwest's wet and temperate forest, while just 30 miles east, over the Continental Divide, begin the vast semiarid prairies of Montana.

Best Time

Spring, summer, and fall, this trail is popular because of its gentle terrain and accessibility from Going-to-the-Sun Road. During hot summer days, the trail remains cool under the huge western red cedars, which act as an umbrella for hikers during inclement weather. During winter, access via cross-country ski or snowshoe is from the winter trailhead at Lake McDonald Lodge and is a 5.8-mile one-way ski. The Trail of the Cedars tends to be icy in winter, so caution is necessary.

Finding the Trail

From Lake McDonald Lodge, drive north on Going-to-the-Sun Road 5.8 miles to the Avalanche

TRAIL USE
Day hiking,
child-friendly,
wheelchair accessible

LENGTH
0.95 mile,
30–45 minutes

VERTICAL FEET
+32'/-32'

DIFFICULTY
1 2 3 4 5

TRAIL TYPE
Loop

SURFACE TYPE
Pavement and
boardwalk

START & END
N48° 40.822'
W113° 49.145'

FEATURES
Flora
Secluded
Birds
Wildlife
Views

FACILITIES
Restroom, Water
Campground
Ranger residence
Shuttle
Picnic area
Phone

Here, you are among the ancients. Count the tree rings on a recently fallen giant next to the boardwalk, and you'll find that these trees were saplings when Thomas Jefferson signed the Declaration of Independence.

Campground, and park in the day-use parking either on your left or along the road in designated day-use parking spots. If taking the free shuttle (available July 1 to Labor Day) from Apgar Transit Center, the trailhead will be 14.7 miles northeast on Going-to-the-Sun Road. Listen for the shuttle driver's announcement for Avalanche Creek. The trailhead sign at the junction of the road and Avalanche Creek will direct you to walk east along the mixed pavement and boardwalk trail.

Trail Description

The trail can be hiked in either direction; this description details a counterclockwise loop beginning on the south side of Avalanche Creek and walking east, where you can glimpse frothy Avalanche Creek with its moss-covered rocks and fishing holes and will encounter a campground, an amphitheater, and a restroom on the south side of the trail.

Camping ▲

Cedars have a fire-resistant quality, thanks to thick bark and moist soils near streams or another body of water. Some trees in this grove are estimated to be nearly 500 years old. Although lightning has started fires nearby, these hardy cedars managed to remain protected. Interpretive signs offer some

Flora 🪶

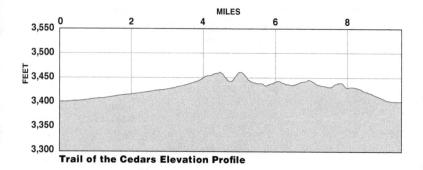

Trail of the Cedars Elevation Profile

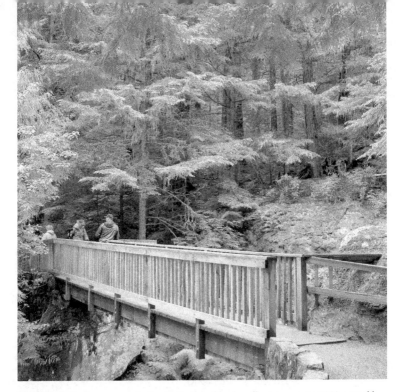

Trail of the Cedars *crosses Avalanche Creek and leads walkers among giant 500-year-old western red cedars.*

insight into flora and fauna. Mostly, however, you'll see fellow hikers, strollers, walkers, and wheelchairs.

Near the halfway point, the trailhead for Avalanche Lake leads east and is clearly marked. Stay on the loop for a magnificent view from a large footbridge at Avalanche Creek gorge. Eons of icy waters have scoured the rock smooth. Beware of the very cold and very fast water. As noted by signs at the Avalanche Lake Trailhead, more people die each year in Glacier from drowning than from any other cause.

The canopy from the cedars and a few hemlocks and cottonwoods is so thick that few shrubs grow here. Notice, however, the fungi and saprophytes (organisms that live on decaying organic matter) that do not rely upon photosynthesis and can thrive in the subdued light.

 Views

Western red cedars, coniferous cypress trees, are among Glacier's 20 tree species, as identified by botanists who also recognize about 90 shrub species in Glacier National Park.

Salish and Kootenai tribes visited this area as a sacred place, calling Lake McDonald the lake of "sacred dancing waters." Evidence indicates the American Indian people visited and fished but didn't live here. Some of these native people wove clothing from tree bark and other fibers.

MILESTONES

►1 0.0   Start from Going-to-the-Sun Road at Avalanche Creek and Avalanche parking area.

►2 0.03 Trail of the Cedars Trailhead

►3 0.28 Where there's a break in the trees, look left and up the cliffs of Mount Cannon and you may see white mountain goats. You'll see Avalanche Creek and get a full view of the giant western red cedars across the creek.

►4 0.46 Just past the Avalanche Lake Trailhead is the Avalanche Creek footbridge, which provides an excellent opportunity for photos of the gorge.

►5 0.6   Benches provide time out to consider the significance of this forest—you can see the massive root system of a windfall cedar. Try counting the rings on another downed cedar that has been sawn apart for trail clearing.

►6 0.9   Cross bridge on Going-to-the-Sun Road.

►7 0.95 Reach Avalanche parking area.

Avalanche Lake Trail

As one of the most popular trails in Glacier, it will probably not be a solitary hike in mid- to late summer. The trail to Avalanche Lake enriches travelers' experiences with varied ecological zones, a mild climb, and a pristine lake fed by several 200-foot waterfalls.

Best Time

The trail, at relatively low elevation, is passable late spring through October. Trail sections are muddy into early July. Skiers tour from Lake McDonald Lodge and up this trail in winter; however, the snow tends to get icy and encrusted with pine needles, making for difficult skiing.

Finding the Trail

From Avalanche Campground area on Going-to-the-Sun Road, hike east past the campground, 0.4 mile on the Trail of the Cedars. The trailhead is 50 feet south of the footbridge over Avalanche Creek. After a dozen steps, you reach a T; the trail veers left/east to the lake.

Trail Description

At the beginning of the hike alongside Avalanche Creek, red rocks—smoothed by the creek as it scours the red argillite rock into a shiny chasm—line the gorge. While it looks inviting, the stream runs high, fast, and frigid—save the wading for the lake. Western red cedars cloak much of the trail's first mile, so look closely for shade-loving orchids and trillium.

TRAIL USE
Day hiking, child-friendly

LENGTH
5.8 miles, 3–4 hours

VERTICAL FEET
±512'

DIFFICULTY
1 **2** 3 4 5

TRAIL TYPE
Out-and-back

SURFACE TYPE
Dirt and gravel

START & END
N48° 40.780'
W113° 49.160'

FEATURES
Lake
Flora
Geologic Interest
Wildlife

FACILITIES
Picnic area
Campgrounds
Ranger-led hikes
Restrooms
Shuttle

 Geologic Interest

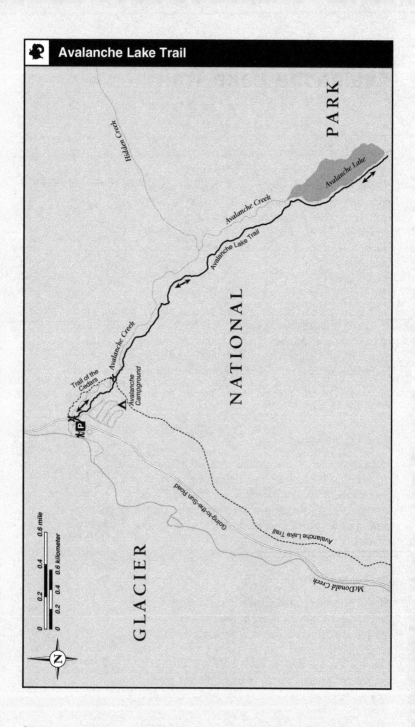

Avalanche Lake Trail

You will come across hulking hulls of ancient western red cedar trees that burned in a lightning fire more than a century ago. Birds, bugs, and rodents thrive in these rotting tree shells. You might catch a glimpse of pileated woodpeckers or hear their laughing call echo through the woods. Northern flying squirrels and red-backed voles join mule deer as well as black bears and grizzly bears thriving here.

Since a massive avalanche in 2011 threw down century-old trees at 1.45 miles, visitors catch significant views of 8,952-foot Mount Cannon and Hidden Creek, as well as a glimpse of the power of an avalanche, which can move snow up to 80 miles per hour, taking trees, rocks, and debris with it. In spring, grizzly bears search the debris for winterkill for necessary protein. You might see mountain goats on Mount Cannon's rocky ledges—the mountain goat kids are quite adept at leaping from ledge to ledge. Binoculars are handy here, yet the goats are visible without them.

The forest changes from heavy cedar and hemlock to more spruce, fir, western larch, and lodgepole pine. The sun finds the forest floor here; thus, more bushes, including huckleberries, flourish. Just before reaching the lake, you come to the lake's outlet, where a logjam plugs the waterway. Continue on the trail; you'll be rewarded with a pebbled beach,

 Wildlife

Nearly 1,000 species of wildflowers are indigenous to Glacier National Park, such as chlorophyll-free Indian pipes, a translucent white flower sometimes called the corpse flower, a shade-loving species.

 Flora

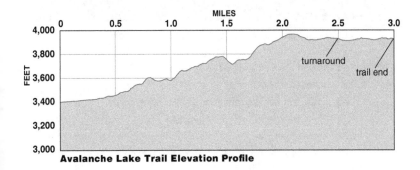

Avalanche Lake Trail Elevation Profile

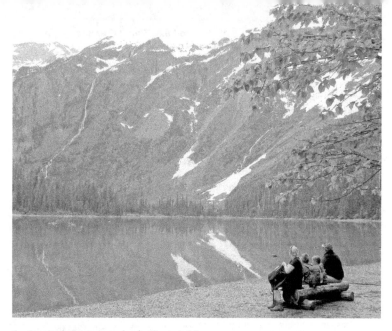

Avalanche Lake *is a popular family picnic hike.*

log benches, and chirping yellow pine chipmunks. Remember that it's illegal to feed the rodents or any wild animal in Glacier.

Avalanche Lake glistens like a gem embedded in the surrounding peaks, striped with waterfalls and dappled with patches of snow. Most people turn around here, but the trail narrows and continues for 0.5 mile to the head of the lake under Little Matterhorn peak.

Lake 〰

🚶	**MILESTONES**	
►1	0.0	Start from Going-to-the-Sun Road at Avalanche Creek and Avalanche parking area.
►2	0.03	Trail of the Cedars Trailhead
►3	0.4	Take left trail at T.
►4	1.45	Downed trees are remnants of 2011 avalanche.
►5	2.14	Outhouses on spur trail to the right
►6	2.2	Avalanche Lake
►7	2.9	Head of Avalanche Lake. Return to trailhead.

Sperry Chalet via Gunsight Pass Trail

The Gunsight Pass Trail to Sperry Chalet climbs from the lush forests of Lake McDonald Valley into a subalpine meadow filled with wildflowers, late-melting snowfields, and curious mountain goats before finally arriving at the chalet. While offering a challenging ascent and descent, the trail exemplifies Glacier's flora zones as it begins amid beargrass, maple, cedar, and hemlock, then climbs through Douglas fir montane with sparse understory and finishes near an alpine meadow at the historic stone-and-log chalet. Glacier National Park sprouts some 1,132 species of vascular plants in two climate zones: Pacific Maritime, as exemplified here along the Sperry Chalet/Gunsight Pass Trail, and Prairie/Arctic, on the east side of the Continental Divide.

Best Time

The trail becomes passable when snow melts, from early July through October. Sperry Chalet is open from early July to early September.

Finding the Trail

From the Lake McDonald Lodge parking lot, walk east across Going-to-the-Sun Road (near the pit toilets). See the large brown sign that reads SPERRY TRAIL. This is the Gunsight Pass Trail—both names are used. Proceed east and pay attention to multiple trail junctions in the first 0.2 mile. You will pass two spur trails to horse concession corrals and the junction with Avalanche Trail to Johns Lake. Continue east to Sperry Chalet on Gunsight Pass Trail.

TRAIL USE
Day hiking, backpacking, horses
LENGTH
12.4 miles, 6–8 hours
VERTICAL FEET
±3,500'
DIFFICULTY
1 2 3 **4** 5
TRAIL TYPE
Out-and-back
SURFACE TYPE
Dirt and gravel
START & END
N48° 37.007'
W113° 52.539'

FEATURES
Flora
Secluded
Geologic Interest
Historic Interest
Wildlife

FACILITIES
Ranger station
Lodging
Restaurants
Stores
Gas
Campgrounds
Backcountry toilets
Backcountry chalet
Water spigot at chalet
    (summer only)
Shuttle

41

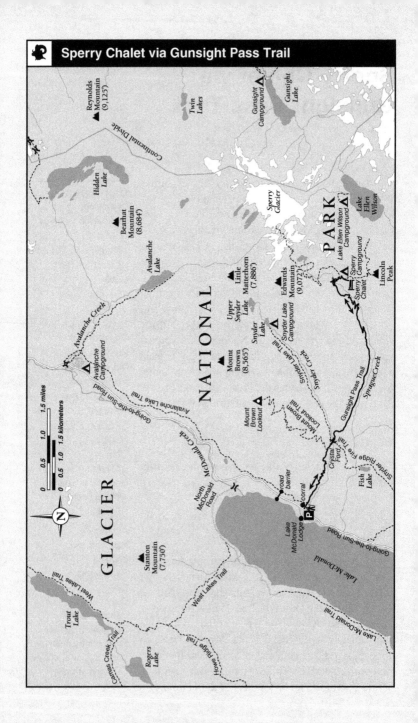

Sperry Chalet via Gunsight Pass Trail

GLACIER

NATIONAL

PARK

Reynolds Mountain (9,125)

Continental Divide

Twin Lakes

Gunsight Campground

Gunsight Lake

Hidden Lake

Bearhat Mountain (8,684)

Avalanche Lake

Sperry Glacier

Lake Ellen Wilson Campground

Lake Ellen Wilson

Little Matterhorn (7,886)

Edwards Mountain (9,072)

Lincoln Peak

Sperry Campground

Sperry Chalet

Avalanche Creek

Upper Snyder Lake

Snyder Lake

Snyder Lake Campground

Snyder Lake Trail

Snyder Creek

Mount Brown (8,565)

Avalanche Campground

Avalanche Lake Trail

Going-to-the-Sun Road

Mount Brown Lookout

Mount Brown Lookout Trail

Gunsight Pass Trail

Sprague Creek

McDonald Creek

Snyder Ridge Fire Trail

Crystal Ford

Fish Lake

0   0.5   1.0   1.5 miles
0   0.5   1.0   1.5 kilometers

North McDonald Road

road barrier

corral

P

Lake McDonald Lodge

Lake McDonald

Going-to-the-Sun Road

Stanton Mountain (7,750)

West Lakes Trail

West Lakes Trail

Lake McDonald Trail

Trout Lake

Camas Creek Trail

Rogers Lake

Howe Ridge Trail

Trail Description

Ten switchbacks climb from 3,200 to 4,200 feet in elevation in the first 1.5 miles, while providing views of roaring Sprague Creek and Lake McDonald. Trail junctions abound, yet the route to Sperry is upward and eastward for almost 2 miles to Crystal Ford, where hikers cross a footbridge and take the left and most-used trail to Sperry.

A switchback along a rock wall of Edwards Mountain ends with a view of Beaver Medicine Falls. A few short switchbacks and a creek crossing later, Sperry Chalet appears on a rocky perch above, right, on the west side of 9,258-foot Gunsight Mountain. The U-shaped glaciated valley sports snow well into July and even August in some years. Look for mountain goats on rocky cliffs. The trail beyond the chalet to Sperry Lake and Sperry Glacier wends left just before you reach the chalet.

Sperry Chalet is worth a visit, even if you are not staying in the historic lodgings. The views into the McDonald Lake Valley reveal the 3,500 feet climbed. The 1914 stone-and-wood structure, built by the Northern Pacific Railway, housed trail-riding tourists. Hotels and backcountry chalets were each a day's horse ride apart, encouraging visitors to travel up to three weeks in America's 10th national park. Today, the chalet, dining hall, and restroom remain

Sperry Chalet (888-345-2649, **sperrychalet.com**), accessible only via trails, opens for lodging and dining July through September and usually books up months in advance. Day hikers can eat lunch in the dining room; reservations are required.

 Wildlife

 Historic Interest

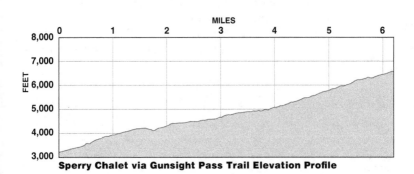

Sperry Chalet via Gunsight Pass Trail Elevation Profile

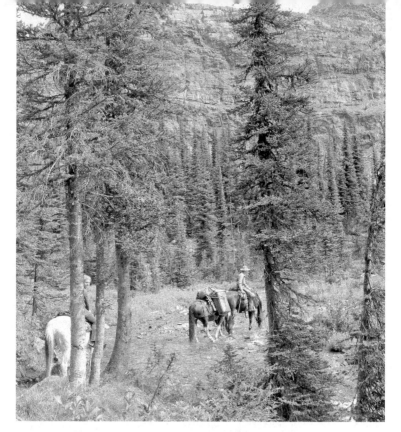

Swan Mountain Outfitters *offers trail rides to Sperry Chalet.*

rustic—no electricity, heat, or running water in the lodgings; headlamps are welcome. The modernized kitchen opens for lunch and dinner to non-lodging guests with reservations. The new restroom uses composting toilets.

The trail sees more than boot prints. Trail riders and pack trains of mules and horses make the

NOTES

College students built this trail in 1902–03 under the direction of Dr. Lyman Sperry of Oberlin College. Sperry led an 1896 party that reached the eponymous glacier. The chalet opened in 1914.

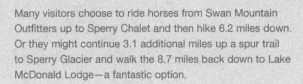

Many visitors choose to ride horses from Swan Mountain
Outfitters up to Sperry Chalet and then hike 6.2 miles down.
Or they might continue 3.1 additional miles up a spur trail
to Sperry Glacier and walk the 8.7 miles back down to Lake
McDonald Lodge—a fantastic option.

trip to Sperry Chalet, packing people and gear up
to the backcountry lodge and returning with some
riders and the chalet's trash. When encountering
stock, step off the trail, talk gently to the animals
and cowboys and cowgirls, and allow the group to
pass. Grizzly and black bears frequent the Sperry/
Gunsight Trail too. Heed trail closure signs.

 Wildlife

☂ MILESTONES

▶1   0.0   Start across Going-to-the-Sun Road from Lake McDonald
Lodge parking area at the SPERRY TRAIL sign.

▶2   0.05   See horse corrals on your left, but proceed east and uphill.

▶3   0.09   Best viewpoint of Lake McDonald, Howe Ridge, and Edwards
Mountain

▶4   0.13   Spur trail heading north to Avalanche Campground

▶5   1.52   Junction with Mount Brown Lookout Trail; continue east
toward Sperry Chalet.

▶6   1.6   Junction with Snyder Lake Trail; take the right/south fork.

▶7   1.73   Bridge over Snyder Creek at Crystal Ford and junction with
Fish Lake Trail; head left/east for Sperry Chalet.

▶8   5.94   Junction with Sperry Glacier Trail

▶9   6.16   Leave Gunsight Pass Trail and take spur trail to Sperry Chalet.

▶10   6.2   Sperry Chalet. Return to trailhead.

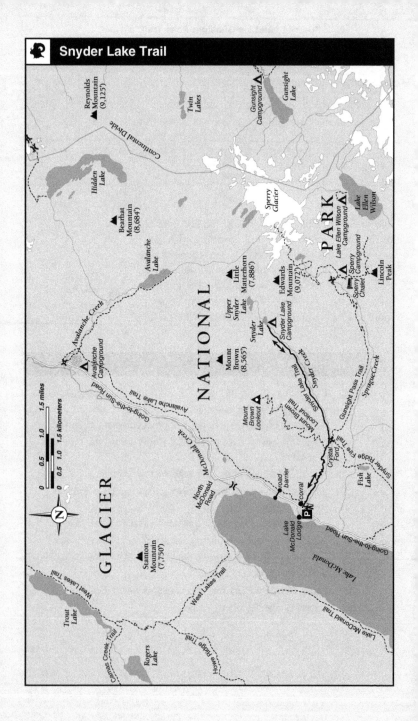

Snyder Lake Trail

Snyder Lake Trail

This family-friendly hike passes through thick timber and past huckleberry bushes to Snyder Lake, filled with an abundance of westslope cutthroat. At the lake, large flat rocks provide the perfect spot for picnics below towering, snow-encrusted cliffs.

Best Time

The lower half of the trail is usually snow-free by April, yet from May to October this trail remains primarily under the protective limbs of shady cedars, pines, tamaracks, and hemlocks. If wind and precipitation dampen the day, this is a good trail for protection from the worst weather—or high temperatures. The final mile is more exposed to the sky.

Finding the Trail

From the Lake McDonald Lodge parking area, look across Going-to-the-Sun Road for the large SPERRY TRAIL sign. This is the Gunsight Pass/Sperry Trail. Note that you will not see a sign for Snyder Lake until you reach the Snyder Lake Trailhead at 1.6 miles. Hike east on the Gunsight Pass/Sperry Trail. Don't be confused by the junction at 1.5 miles for Mount Brown Lookout Trail—remain on the main trail until you see the Snyder Lake signpost; the Snyder Lake Trail forks left from Sperry Trail at mile 1.6. If you miss this junction, you will find yourself at the Snyder Creek footbridge and a stock crossing called Crystal Ford—you've gone 0.2 mile too far.

TRAIL USE
Day hiking, child-friendly, horses

LENGTH
8.4 miles, 4–6 hours

VERTICAL FEET
+2,146'/-2,146'

DIFFICULTY
1 2 **3** 4 5

TRAIL TYPE
Out-and-back

SURFACE TYPE
Dirt

START & END
N48° 37.007'
W113° 52.539'

FEATURES
Flora
Secluded
Wildlife
Views
Lake
Swimming
Fishing

FACILITIES
Lodge
Camp store
Campground
Shuttle service

Trail Description

Lake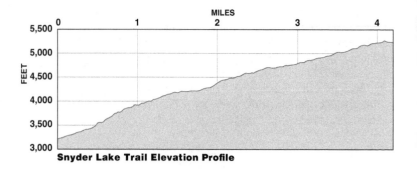
The lovely green-blue lake at the end of the 4.2 miles is worth the initial 1,000 feet of climbing. The trail's umbrella of western red cedar, western hemlock, and deciduous tamarack trees shelters the trail so that during the climb, you're in the shade. Three of the switchbacks provide viewpoints of Lake McDonald and Howe Ridge to the west, snow-flecked Lincoln Peak to the east, and Snyder Creek rushing well below the trail. Swan Mountain Outfitters leads trail rides on this route to nearby Sperry Chalet and pack trains of mules or horses to supply the backcountry chalet and work crews. Be sure to step off the trail, but talk to the wrangler, guests, and livestock so you do not spook the steeds.

Views

As you climb, notice how the cedars give way to lodgepole pine and significantly more understory: bushes of huckleberry, elderberry, and strawberry, all of which are bear favorites. Make plenty of noise as you hike to ward off bears. It's now an easier climb past the Mount Brown Lookout Trail junction. A short walk later, you'll meet the junction for Snyder Lake Trail, so veer left. If you descend to a creek, footbridge, and stock crossing called Crystal Ford, you've gone too far. From the trail junction, it's 2.6 miles to the lake among open-forest, marshy areas where ferns

Flora

Wildlife

Snyder Lake Trail Elevation Profile

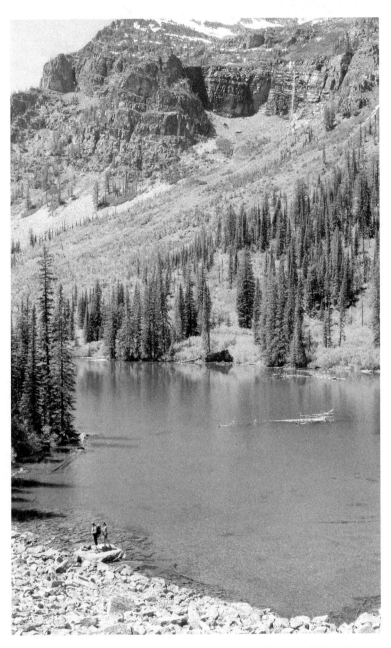

Snyder Lake is named *for Glacier's first hotelier, George Snyder, who built his hotel in 1895 on the shore of Lake McDonald.*

and lots of wildflowers, including beargrass, dominate the trailside. The lodgepole pines sport moss called old man's beard, which hangs from the limbs like 2-foot-long, lime-green whiskers.

Notice the avalanche paths sweeping down from the shoulder of Mount Brown on your left. In some places, the trees have been snapped off 25 feet high as snow and ice sped down chutes in winter and early spring. You'll cross a rock slide of lichen-covered limestone, at which point you are only 0.4 mile from the lake. A hitching post on the left might have saddle horses tethered to it. The footbridge across Snyder Creek is a few steps away. The lake's three campsites, food-prep area, and food-hanging pole, plus a new outhouse, are near the foot of the lake just beyond the footbridge.

Camping

Follow the thinning trail to several large, flat rocks just offshore—perfect for picnics or for casting a fly to the westslope cutthroat trout residing here. Several waterfalls splash down toward this cirque-enclosed loch. Upper Snyder Lake, of similar size to the main lake, is a trail-less scramble and another 0.25 mile northeast. Fall colors are spectacular evergreen, red, and gold around the lake and below the Little Matterhorn peak.

Autumn Colors

🚶 MILESTONES

▶1 0.0   Start from Going-to-the-Sun Road at Lake McDonald Lodge's parking area and the SPERRY TRAIL sign.

▶2 0.05 See horse corrals on your left, but proceed east and uphill.

▶3 0.09 Best viewpoint of Lake McDonald, Howe Ridge, and Edwards Mountain

▶4 0.13 Spur trail heading north to Avalanche Campground

▶5 1.52 Junction with Mount Brown Lookout

▶6 1.6   Snyder Lake Trail junction

▶7 1.63 View of Edwards Mountain

▶8 3.8   Cross a rock slide.

▶9 4.18 Hitching post and footbridge to lake, campsites, and outhouse

▶10 4.2 Snyder Lake. Return to trailhead.

Snyder Lake is one of 131 named lakes in the park and is surrounded by Mount Brown, the Little Matterhorn, and Edwards Mountain—just beyond the Little Matterhorn is Avalanche Lake, another Top Trail (Trail 2), and above, Sperry Glacier. Snyder Lake is exceedingly clear—you can clearly see the lake bed 30 feet down, thanks to minimal plankton—and water temperatures are around 50°F in summer.

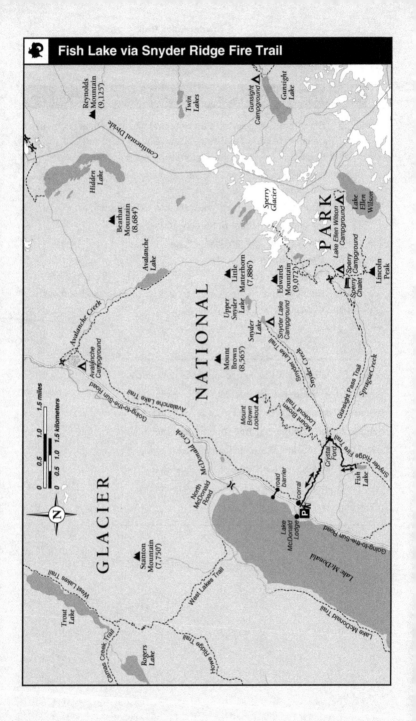

Fish Lake via Snyder Ridge Fire Trail

This lovely wooded hike through alder, hemlock, Douglas fir, lodgepole, and the occasional western red cedar leads to a quiet lake surrounded by a healthy forest. In fall, the colors from tamarack, a deciduous conifer, illuminate the trail in golden hues, while Rocky Mountain maple leaves add deep red to the forest. Fish Lake attracts the occasional fisherman who has packed in a float tube and fly rod. Fishing from shore is doable, although trees line much of the shore, requiring some accurate back-casting to avoid hooking the foliage.

Best Time

The trail remains mostly shaded and therefore is an excellent choice for a rainy late-spring hike in May, as well as hot summer days. The trail is usually snow-free by late May, although sections can be damp to wet through June.

Finding the Trail

From the Lake McDonald Lodge parking area, walk east across Going-to-the-Sun Road (near the pit toilets). Look for the large brown SPERRY TRAIL sign. This is the Gunsight Pass Trail, which accesses the Snyder Ridge Fire Trail to Fish Lake. Note that you will not see a sign for Fish Lake for almost 2 trail miles, until just after the Crystal Ford footbridge.

TRAIL USE
Day hiking, child-friendly

LENGTH
5.8 miles, 3–4 hours

VERTICAL FEET
±1,000'

DIFFICULTY
1 **2** 3 4 5

TRAIL TYPE
Out-and-back

SURFACE TYPE
Dirt and gravel

START & END
N48° 37.007'
W113° 52.539'

FEATURES
Flora
Secluded
Geologic Interest
Historic Interest
Wildlife
Lake
Fishing

FACILITIES
Lodging, Restaurants
Stores, Gas
Interpretive center
Campgrounds
Shuttle

Trail Description

The trail follows the route toward Sperry Chalet, initially passing the horse corrals' spur trails and a junction with the trail to Johns Lake before climbing a series of switchbacks. Don't take any northbound trails. At several switchbacks, you can look to the south for views of Snyder Creek and Lake McDonald. These will be nearly the only broad views on this hike because the dense forest cloaks the peaks. The same thick overstory, however, protects the trail from wind, rain, and hot sun. You may encounter pack trains and trail rides; yield to the mules and horses by stepping off the trail. When upper elevation treks are impassable due to snow, the hike to Fish Lake is generally snow-free.

After passing the junctions with Mount Brown Lookout Trail at mile 1.52 and Snyder Lake Trail at 1.6, your route zips down to Crystal Ford. The footbridge over Snyder Creek provides a great photo op over the frothy green creek. After crossing Snyder Creek, the trail splits. Take the right fork uphill toward Fish Lake. This is the Snyder Ridge Fire Trail.

There's a brief climb before the trail flattens out and cruises into an old-growth forest where the trail is cushioned with pine needles. Look for black-tailed deer, spruce grouse, and pileated woodpecker.

No fishing license or permit is needed to fish inside Glacier National Park. Some rivers, streams, and lakes are closed for fish spawning, eagle nesting, or other seasonal events. Check with the park regarding fishing regulations.

Wildlife

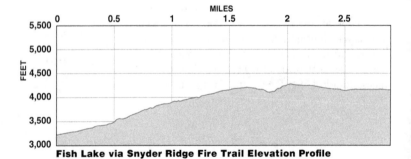

Fish Lake via Snyder Ridge Fire Trail Elevation Profile

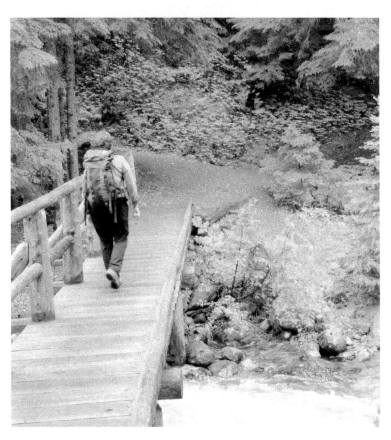

Glacier has *some 700 lakes, ponds, marshes, and bogs—wetlands that provide habitat for six amphibian species, including the long-toed salamander, which has a chartreuse stripe down its back.*

The quarter-mile-long lake is home to numerous waterfowl, such as the common merganser, the common goldeneye, frogs, and songbirds. The yellow water lily floating here has large yellow flowers and 6- to 8-inch lily pads. Local American Indians used the water lily seeds, grinding them into flour for baking. If you venture around to the south side of the lake, a brushy route, you can see Mount Brown and its lookout to the north.

 Lake

 Flora

 Historic Interest

MILESTONES

►1	0.0	Start from Going-to-the-Sun Road at Lake McDonald Lodge's parking area and the SPERRY TRAIL sign.
►2	0.05	See horse corrals on your left, but proceed east and uphill.
►3	0.09	Best viewpoint of Lake McDonald, Howe Ridge, and Edwards Mountain
►4	0.13	Spur trail heading north to Avalanche Campground
►5	1.52	Junction with Mount Brown Lookout Trail
►6	1.6	Snyder Lake Trail junction
►7	1.72	Bridge over Snyder Creek at Crystal Ford and junction with Fish Lake Trail; head right/west to Fish Lake on Snyder Ridge Fire Trail.
►7	2.9	Fish Lake. Return to trailhead.

NOTES

Snyder Ridge is named for the first hotelier to build lodgings on Lake McDonald, George Snyder, whose 1895 two-story stopover proved insufficient for the number of visitors. He soon built a larger hotel on the site of today's Lake McDonald Lodge.

OPTIONS

The Snyder Ridge Fire Trail can be hiked through to Going-to-the-Sun Road. This would make for an additional 3 miles to Lincoln Lake Trailhead at Going-to-the-Sun Road, requiring a shuttle.

Mount Brown Lookout Trail

As one of the most challenging hikes in the park, the constant uphill to the Mount Brown Lookout tests even the fittest of hikers. The trip back downhill scrunches toes into boots and wearies the knees. Despite the difficult ascent and descent, the trail rewards hikers with views of Lake McDonald and Fish Lake below, as well as Heavens Peak, Mount Vaught, McPartland Mountain, Sperry Glacier, and more. Plus, the lookout itself is a remarkable feat of construction, here on a windswept rock outcrop along the south shoulder of Mount Brown. The materials for the clapboard building were hauled up to the site via mule pack trains and backpacks in 1929. Extra water and hiking poles make the trip more enjoyable.

Best Time

The trail is mostly snow-free by late June; however, deadfall makes a challenging trail even more difficult until trail crews clear it, usually by early July. Because the trail climbs 4,250 feet in elevation and the latter third is above the treeline, it's best to hike early in the day.

Finding the Trail

From the Lake McDonald Lodge parking lot, walk east across Going-to-the-Sun Road (near the pit toilets). See the large brown SPERRY TRAIL sign; this is the Gunsight Pass Trail—both names are used. Proceed east on the trail and pay attention to multiple trail junctions in the first 0.2 mile. You will pass two

TRAIL USE
Day hiking

LENGTH
10.1 miles, 5–8 hours

VERTICAL FEET
±4,250'

DIFFICULTY
1 2 3 4 **5**

TRAIL TYPE
Out-and-back

SURFACE TYPE
Dirt and gravel

START & END
N48° 37.007'
W113° 52.539'

FEATURES
Flora
Secluded
Geologic Interest
Historic Interest
Wildlife
Views

FACILITIES
Ranger station
Lodging
Restaurants
Stores
Gas
Interpretive center
Campgrounds
Shuttle

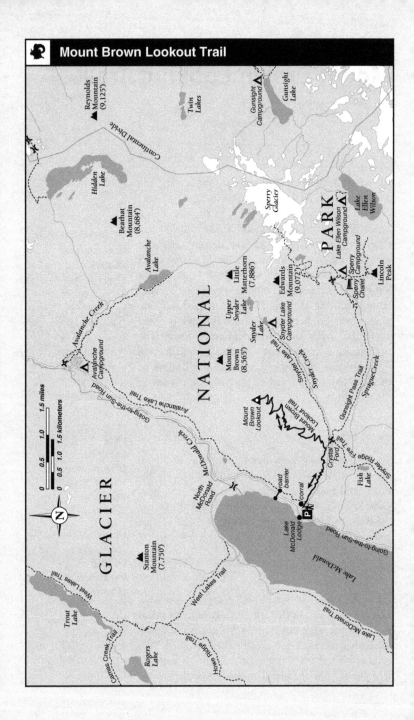

spur trails to horse concession corrals and the junction with Avalanche Trail to Johns Lake. Continue east to Mount Brown Lookout Trailhead at mile 1.5.

Trail Description

After the initial upward hike through the hemlock- and cedar-forested Sperry Chalet/Gunsight Pass Trail, the Mount Brown Lookout Trail climbs mercilessly for a mile. Trees shade much of the next 1.5 miles, where beargrass and huckleberry join the understory growth. Four viewpoints along the route include spectacular observation points of 9,072-foot Edwards Mountain at a rocky outcrop switchback, which tops the steepest section of the trail. The trail traces back into the trees, where you catch glimpses of Lake McDonald below. At 6,612-feet elevation, there's another viewpoint of Edwards. Small groves of Engelmann spruce on windy ridges are separated by subalpine meadows and dwarf subalpine fir.

The final push to the lookout crosses a plateau cloaked in yellow glacier lilies, which appear in the melting snowfield usually in mid-July. Keep an eye out for *Ursus arctos horribilis*—grizzly bears gnaw on lily bulbs; you may see where one has dredged up

The peak is named for the solicitor general of the Chicago and Alton Railroad, William Brown, who made the first ascent of the mountain in 1894.

 Flora

Views

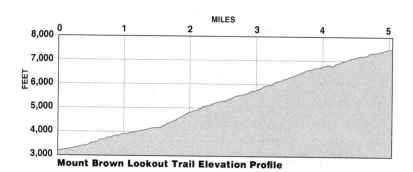
Mount Brown Lookout Trail Elevation Profile

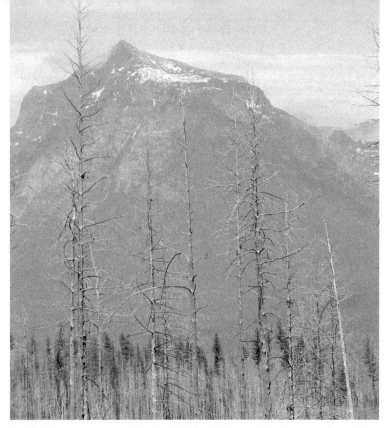

Mount Brown, *viewed here from across McDonald Valley, sports a fire lookout on its right shoulder 1,100 feet below the summit.*

the soil. Mountain goats clippity-clop through here, too, in their never-ending search for lichens, moss, grass, herbs, and sedges. Look out over the Edwards Mountain and the Little Matterhorn area, and you might see a bald eagle circling below. Bald eagles subsist mostly on fish but will hunt other waterbirds, such as ducks and geese, and are opportunists when it comes to carrion.

Wildlife

The two-story, 14-foot-square lookout included few comforts: a wood-burning stove, a cot, a wood table and chairs, cupboards, and a centrally located fire finder, the alidade, mounted on a wood stand. The alidade helped the fire scout locate a distant object or fire on a map by employing line of

Historic Interest

> As an atmospheric discharge of electricity, lightning can be
> fatal to park visitors, who should seek shelter from lightning
> storms. "Cold stroke" lightning sends high-voltage, short-
> duration strikes. "Hot stroke" lightning delivers lower voltage
> over a longer duration. About one in five strokes hit the ground.

CAUTION

sight using a rotating bezel. While hikers can access the catwalk around the lookout, the building is locked and shuttered.

The peak's summit is another 1,100 feet above the lookout. Hiking beyond the lookout requires technical climbing gear and skills to access rocky realms.

Now listed on the National Register of Historic Places, the 1928 lookout housed fire scouts until 1971. In 1999, it was refurbished, although it's not used as a lookout.

MILESTONES

▶1 0.0   Start across Going-to-the-Sun Road from Lake McDonald Lodge parking area at the SPERRY TRAIL sign.

▶2 0.05 Spur trail to horse concession corral heads left/north; hike uphill and east.

▶3 0.09 Another spur trail to horse concession corral heads left/north; hike uphill and east.

▶4 1.52 Junction with Mount Brown Lookout Trail; take the left/north trail toward the lookout.

▶5 5.05 Mount Brown Lookout. Return to trailhead.

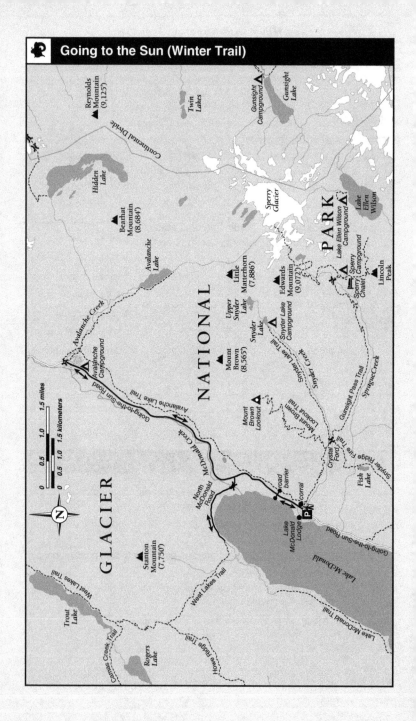

Going to the Sun (Winter Trail)

Reynolds Mountain (9,125')

Continental Divide

Twin Lakes

Gunsight Campground

Gunsight Lake

Hidden Lake

Sperry Glacier

Beartaht Mountain (8,684')

PARK

Lake Ellen Wilson

Avalanche Lake

Little Matterhorn (7,886')

Edwards Mountain (9,072')

Sperry Campground

Lincoln Peak

Upper Snyder Lake

NATIONAL

Sperry Chalet

Avalanche Creek

Snyder Lake

Snyder Lake Campground

Snyder Lake Trail

Mount Brown (8,565')

Snyder Creek

Avalanche Campground

Avalanche Lake Trail

Gunsight Pass Trail

Sprague Creek

Mount Brown Lookout

Mount Brown Lookout Trail

Going-to-the-Sun Road

Snyder Ridge Fire Trail

North McDonald Road

McDonald Creek

Crystal Ford

Fish Lake

GLACIER

0   0.5   1.0   1.5 miles

0   0.5 1.0 1.5 kilometers

N

Stanton Mountain (7,750')

road barrier

Corral

Lake McDonald Lodge

P

Going-to-the-Sun Road

West Lakes Trail

Lake McDonald

Lake McDonald Trail

Trout Lake

Canas Creek Trail

Rogers Lake

Howe Ridge Trail

Going-to-the-Sun (Winter Trail)

Winter in Glacier is a magical time when few visitors share the trails. While it may seem that the park is in hibernation, many subnivean creatures are active under the 5 feet of annual snowfall. Deer, beavers, bald eagles, and the rare and beautiful harlequin duck thrive in brumal solitude. Winter conditions may exist from early November through June.

Best Time

The trail becomes skiable late November through March, depending upon snow depth and conditions. If the trail becomes icy, the difficulty level increases; the trip takes longer as well.

Finding the Trail

From Lake McDonald Lodge parking lot, walk south on the sidewalks to Going-to-the-Sun Road and find the road-closure barriers. Put skis or snowshoes on, and follow the road north toward Avalanche Campground. The entire trail is on the snowed-in road.

Trail Description

Initially, the ski trail along Going-to-the-Sun Road is a combination of rolling hills and long, flat sections. At the junction, adventurers continue north along Going-to-the-Sun Road, which offers fantastic observation points for the partially frozen and frothy McDonald Creek. The observation point for McDonald Falls and Sacred Dancing Cascade

TRAIL USE
Skiing, snowshoeing, youth-friendly

LENGTH
16.8 miles, 2–6 hours

VERTICAL FEET
±234'

DIFFICULTY
1 2 3 4 5 (depending on iciness of trail)

TRAIL TYPE
Out-and-back

SURFACE TYPE
Snow and ice

START & END
N48° 37.007'
W113° 52.539'

FEATURES
Secluded
Geologic Interest
Historic Interest
Wildlife
Views

FACILITIES
Phone
Campgrounds

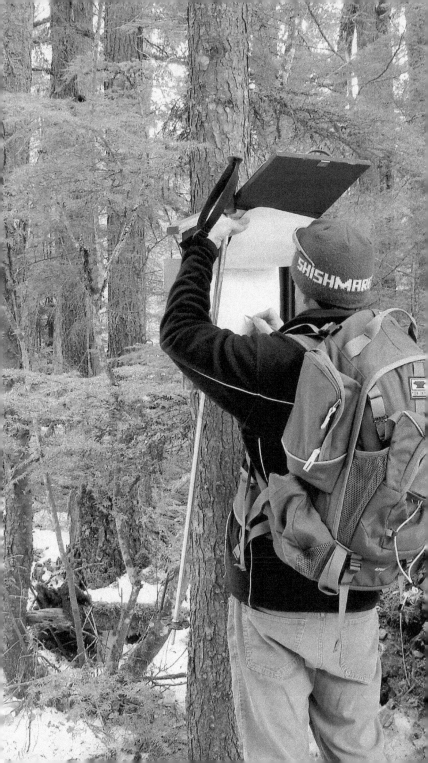

may be slippery and dangerous. As you continue north, you pass the places where the creek is close to the trail. It's here that harlequin ducks luxuriate in the frigid waters of wintry April after their 600-mile migration from the Pacific Coast. You might encounter researchers banding, counting, and documenting the rare waterfowl's habits.

 Views

As you travel, you will catch glimpses of 8,565-foot Mount Brown, topped with a shuttered fire lookout, and even the 8,000-foot Garden Wall. Much of the forest of evergreens is dense and dark yet offers protection from weather. This is also where you might glimpse deer, porcupine, and moose. Know that reclusive badgers, Canadian lynx, and mountain lions also reside here.

Wildlife

The ski tracks are made from snowshoes, kick-and-glide skiers, and the occasional winter walker (snowmobiles are forbidden). The park rangers ask that visitors snowshoe, ski, or walk on separate tracks to avoid crushing the other sport's tracks—side-by-side routes in snow. Some experienced skiers skate ski when conditions are favorable for crust cruising. Check your watch—sunset at winter solstice is at 4:45 p.m., and only the moon and your headlamp will illuminate the trail if you're out after sunset.

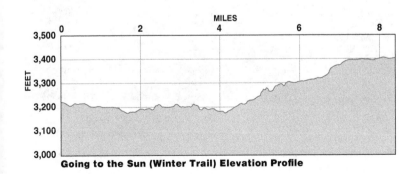

Going to the Sun (Winter Trail) Elevation Profile

Note: Many skiers and snowshoers do a portion of the trail and often turn back at the falls overlook.

Though this route does not traipse upon avalanche-prone territory, it's a good idea to check weather, snow, and avalanche conditions. Skiers can access slopes near this winter trail that might present dangerous snowslides. Find local avalanche conditions at **flatheadavalanche.org.** Two outfitters provide snowshoe and ski guide service and gear rentals: Glacier Adventure Guides (406-892-2173) and Izaak Walton Inn (406-888-5700). Izaak Walton Inn also offers year-round lodging. None of the Glacier Park lodges operate in winter; however, many lodging options are available in nearby West Glacier, Whitefish, and Kalispell: **explorewhitefish.com.**

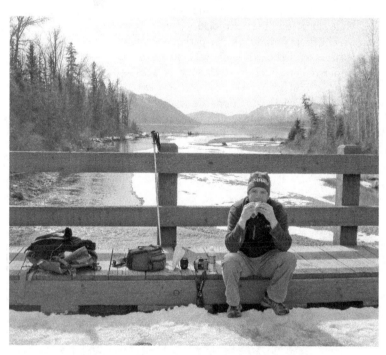

Spring skiing and picnicking *on the bridge over McDonald Creek provides views of McDonald Lake during a March thaw.*

🚶 MILESTONES

►1	0.0	Start from the Lake McDonald Lodge parking lot and head north on Going-to-the-Sun Road.
►2	0.5	At the road barrier, put on skis or snowshoes, and ski on the road.
►3	1.46	At the road junction, take the left/west spur on North Lake McDonald Road ski trail, which travels around the lake's northern and western shore, an out-and-back route.
►4	2.9	Turn around at the trail junction.
►5	4.36	Return to road junction and continue north on Going-to-the-Sun Road.
►6	8.4	Turn around at Avalanche Campground.

About 200 pairs of harlequin ducks nest annually in Glacier, producing 25% of Montana's harlequin chicks. The "painted" ducks, considered a species of concern, thrive in turbulent whitewater. A drake is called a lord, and a hen is called a lady.

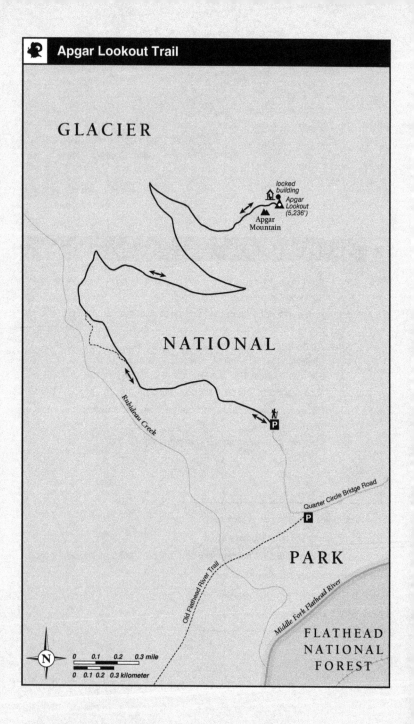

Apgar Lookout Trail

GLACIER

locked building

Apgar Lookout (5,236')

Apgar Mountain

NATIONAL

Rabideau Creek

Quarter Circle Bridge Road

PARK

Old Flathead River Trail

Middle Fork Flathead River

FLATHEAD NATIONAL FOREST

N

| 0 | 0.1 | 0.2 | 0.3 mile |
| 0 | 0.1 | 0.2 | 0.3 kilometer |

Apgar Lookout Trail

Tall western hemlock, aspen, and brush shade the trail as it gently climbs, inviting families to explore the forest, which is prime habitat for birds. In fact, on summer mornings, mountain bluebirds, rufous hummingbirds, and western tanagers join a songbird serenade.

Best Time

This trail is snow-free earlier than most trails in the West Glacier area because much of the route traverses a south-facing mountainside, where snow melts late May to early June most years. Because of the 2003 fires, the trail is now exposed to the elements, so on hot summer days, it's best to hike in the morning.

Finding the Trail

From the West Glacier entrance station, head north about 0.25 mile, and look for the large brown sign with white letters that says HORSEBACK RIDES, GLACIER INSTITUTE, APGAR LOOKOUT. Turn left/west, and follow the paved road to a Y and another large sign pointing right to APGAR LOOKOUT TRAIL, HORSE RENTALS. (As the sign indicates, a left turn takes you to the Glacier Institute's camp.) As you head right, you will arrive at the horse concession; stay left, as the sign to Quarter Circle Bridge indicates. The paved road becomes gravel as you drive the 0.5 mile to Quarter Circle Bridge—cross the one-lane wooden bridge cautiously as rafting parties and bridge-jumping swimmers clog the area. The gravel road narrows to one lane for the next 1.4

TRAIL USE
Day hiking, child-friendly

LENGTH
7.2 miles, 4–6 hours

VERTICAL FEET
±1,989'

DIFFICULTY
1 2 **3** 4 5

TRAIL TYPE
Out-and-back

SURFACE TYPE
Dirt and gravel

START & END
N48° 30.270'
W114° 01.264'

FEATURES
Birds
Flora
Secluded
Geologic Interest
Historic Interest
Wildlife
Views
Photo opportunity

FACILITIES
Ranger station
Lodging
Restaurants
Grocery store, Gas
Gift/gear shop
Horse outfitter
Rafting outfitters
Interpretive center
Campgrounds

The Roberts Fire that burned Apgar Mountain was one of several fires that burned 136,000 acres of Glacier National Park in 2003.

miles to the Apgar Lookout Trailhead. As you enter the parking area, look to your left for the trail sign, which lets you know the lookout is 3.6 miles away.

Trail Description

This trail begins on an old logging road wide enough for hikers to walk side by side for half a mile. As the route begins to climb, hikers will notice trailside groups of western red cedars that survived fire; it's interesting that all other vegetation and trees for acres burned in the 2003 fires. Meadow areas reveal several small, marshy ponds, each about an acre or two in size—perfect moose habitat. Ahead on the right looms Apgar Mountain; part of the trail is visible as it switchbacks up the south side of the mountain.

Look for elk, mule deer, and moose below, near the trees and marshy meadows. You might hear a blue grouse ruffling before you see it. This is also home to the American marten, a tan to dark-brown, vole-eating predator of the weasel family. You may also hear and see trains on the old Great Northern Railway route, just outside the park and along the Middle Fork of the Flathead River. The tracks host several trains, including the twice-daily Amtrak and

Flora

Wildlife

Birds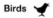

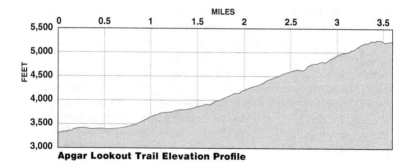

Apgar Lookout Trail Elevation Profile

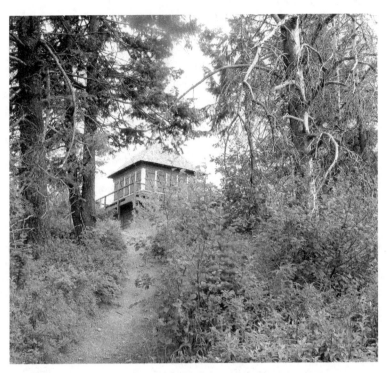

The shuttered Apgar Lookout's *accessible deck provides outstanding views into the Lake McDonald valley.*

> Check the trail status with the park entrance station: Quarter Circle Bridge Road is closed and gated in late fall until the snow melts in late spring.

multiple daily Burlington Northern–Santa Fe cargo trains. It's part of the West Glacier area outside the park, hemmed by the Middle Fork and dotted with a few homes, lodgings, and eateries.

The unmanned lookout tower is actually just east of Apgar Mountain's summit and about 200 feet below the peak. The 1929 Apgar Lookout is listed on the National Register of Historic Places. A hitching rail, two pit toilets, and communication towers are nearby. Hikers can climb the lookout's stairs for views from the wraparound porch of the two-story,

 Historic Interest

Apgar Lookout, along with the village, peak, and range, were named after homesteader Milo B. Apgar, who arrived in 1892 from Maine.

Views

wood-framed building, which is shuttered and locked. The National Park Service maintains a webcam at the lookout. For a view from the top, as well as current temperature and humidity, see **nps .gov/glac/photosmultimedia/webcams.htm**.

Mountaintop rewards include views to the north and northwest of Lake McDonald, the Garden Wall, the Belton Hills, and the Lewiston Range. Beyond spreads the North Fork region of Glacier, about 50 miles away. The viewpoint provides a striking scene of patchwork burns, denuded timber, and green forest, all remnants of the 2003 Roberts Fire.

MILESTONES

▶1 0.0 Start from the parking lot and trailhead, hiking west through tall timbers and wildflower-strewn meadows.

▶2 0.5 Trail narrows and climbs into a meadow and marshy ponds area thick with ungulates such as moose, elk, and deer. Listen for songbirds.

▶3 1.4 Trail begins the long switchbacks up Apgar Mountain.

▶4 3.6 Apgar Lookout. Return to trailhead.

Huckleberry Mountain Lookout Trail

While the lower portion of Huckleberry Mountain remains mostly shaded year-round, the upper half of the trail explodes in wildflowers in late June and July. The trail is initially flat for a mile and then climbs gently and steadily nearly all the rest of the way, providing new views each mile.

Best Time

The trail is damp but mostly snow-free by mid-June; however, two snowfield crossings in the final mile may require hiking poles and crampons, depending upon how icy and steep the conditions become. Unless you're hiking with a large group, avoid this trail after Labor Day due to the many grizzly bears seeking huckleberries and other forage.

Finding the Trail

From the Camas Creek Entrance, drive east 4 miles to the six parking spaces on the south side of the road. From Apgar, drive west on Camas Creek Road, and drive 6 miles to the parking area, which is between two overlooks: McGee Meadow Overlook is 0.2 mile east of the trailhead; Camas Creek Overlook is 2 miles west of the trailhead on the north side of the road. A large brown sign indicates the Huckleberry Lookout. The trail leads south from the south edge of the parking area.

TRAIL USE
Day hiking

LENGTH
12.0 miles, 5–7 hours

VERTICAL FEET
±2,706'

DIFFICULTY
1 2 **3** 4 5

TRAIL TYPE
Out-and-back

SURFACE TYPE
Dirt, gravel, and pine needles

START & END
N48° 35.794'
W114° 02.307'

FEATURES
Flora
Secluded
Geologic Interest
Historic Interest
Wildlife
Views

FACILITIES
Lookout
Stock ramp

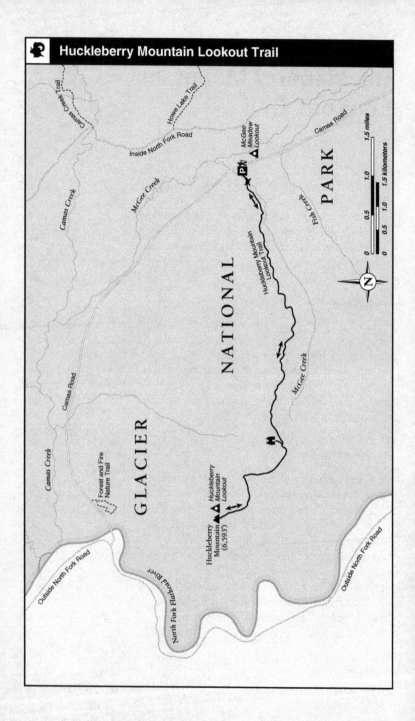

Trail Description

Hikers and trail riders frequent the Huckleberry Mountain Lookout Trail and find that the wooded and damp first mile can be buggy. The route crosses several streamlets, most of which have both a small footbridge and a stock crossing nearby. If you've reached a wide stream crossing where it is evident that horses stepped through the water, you probably missed the correct passageway. Retrace 25 steps and find the footpath to a plank footbridge. The high water table here contributes to the nearby McGee Meadow fen, a peatland with groundwater flowing throughout the marshy area. The rare bog lemming makes its home here among the cotton grass, buckler fern, and bladderwort, an insect-devouring plant. The floating bladder's hair trigger inflates when bumped by an insect, and then the bladderwort consumes the insect using digestive enzymes.

As the trail wends through lodgepole pine and hemlock, notice delicate orchids, such as the fairy slipper orchid, and numerous fungi and ferns. The trail bed is cushioned by pine needles silencing footsteps. At 2.5 miles, trees thin and allow views below of McGee Creek valley and above to the Apgar Range. Unlike much of the park, this area has thick stands of healthy lodgepole pine, thanks to

Famous writers Edward Abbey and Doug Peacock manned Glacier's lookouts—Abbey at Numa in 1975, and Peacock at Huckleberry and Scalplock between 1976 and 1984.

 Flora

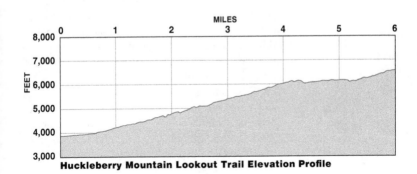

Huckleberry Mountain Lookout Trail Elevation Profile

Huckleberry Mountain Lookout *provides the fire scout—and visiting hikers—excellent views of the North Fork of the Flathead River valley.*

Wildlife

Wildflowers

Views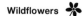

1967 fires that burned the area, allowing new trees to sprout. The wildflowers and berries in the alpine bowl attract songbirds, bees, and bears among the fireweed, Indian paintbrush, beargrass, and red currants. Once you reach the notch at 4.2 miles, you can take a quick spur route right/northeast for 200 yards to a view of the lookout; however, the trail heads the opposite way, left and around the north side of Huckleberry Mountain. You won't see the lookout until you are on the final jaunt along the grassy ridgeline of the peak. Note that in May and June, two snowfields create hazardous travel at the notch and again just below the lookout.

Outstanding views of the North Fork's peaks and into Canada are camera-worthy. You can see why the lookout is still manned: Evidence of the 2001 Moose Fire and 2003 Roberts Fire Complex can be seen in the patchwork of dead standing trees next to thick, green, untouched trees.

NOTES

The trail's namesake, the huckleberry, is a local delicacy. Purple berries hang on 1- to 3-foot-tall bushes late July through September, depending on elevation. Two varieties grow in Glacier: common huckleberry and low huckleberry. Their relative in the heath family (Ericaceae), the fool's huckleberry, grows 7 feet tall, has capsules instead of berries, smells skunky, and is considered poisonous.

⚐ MILESTONES

▶1   0.0   Start from Camas Creek Road, 6 miles west of Apgar.

▶2   4.2   At the notch, follow the trail heading left/west to the lookout, or turn uphill and right/northeast for 200 yards for a view of the lookout.

▶3   5.5   At saddle, follow the ridgeline trail.

▶4   6.0   Huckleberry Mountain Lookout. Return to parking area.

Huckleberry is one of four fire lookouts in Glacier that remain in service, along with Numa, Scalplock, and Loneman Lookouts. Huckleberry Lookout has twice burned down and been rebuilt.

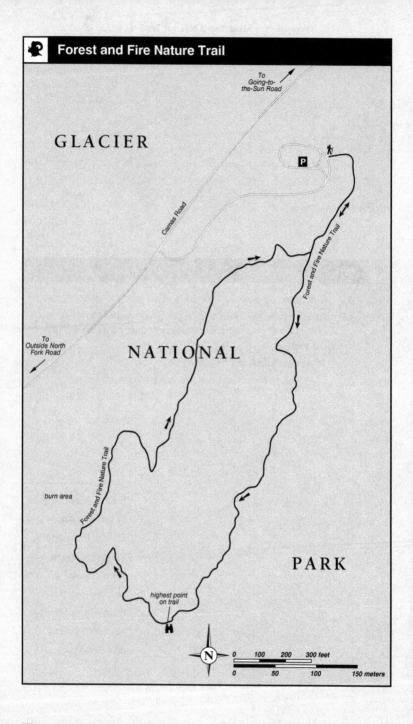

Forest and Fire Nature Trail

GLACIER

To
Going-to-
the-Sun Road

Camas Road

P

Forest and Fire Nature Trail

To
Outside North
Fork Road

NATIONAL

Forest and Fire Nature Trail

burn area

PARK

highest point
on trail

N

| 0 | 100 | 200 | 300 feet |
| 0 | 50 | 100 | 150 meters |

Forest and Fire Nature Trail
(formerly Huckleberry Nature Trail)

As the premier trail for exploring wildfire and recovery, this family-friendly loop was initially created to explain the 1967 Huckleberry Mountain Fire. In the 2001 Moose Fire, the trail and 71,000 acres burned. Formerly called the Huckleberry Nature Trail, the Forest and Fire Nature Trail is an expansive example of forest regeneration. Note that some older trail maps list the original trail name.

Best Time

The trail is hikable nearly year-round, although it is snow-covered and possibly icy in the winter months. From March through October, the trail varies from dry to muddy or mixed snow and debris.

Finding the Trail

From the Camas Creek park entrance area, 500 feet beyond the vehicle pull-off and park entrance sign, the parking area is on the south side of Camas Creek Road and is marked. The parking area is about 10 miles from Apgar on Camas Creek Road. The paved parking area has six parking spots, plus one handicapped spot. Note that after the initial 50 yards, the trail is not wide enough for a wheelchair or a stroller or wheeled jogger.

Trail Description

The view of Huckleberry Mountain, from the trailhead looking south, is thick with regrowth where most of the scorched timber has fallen, although a

TRAIL USE
Day hiking, child-friendly

LENGTH
1.0 mile,
30 minutes–1 hour

VERTICAL FEET
±42'

DIFFICULTY
1 2 3 4 5

TRAIL TYPE
Balloon

SURFACE TYPE
Dirt and gravel

START & END
N48° 37.470'
W114° 07.770'

FEATURES
Flora
Birds
Secluded
Geologic Interest
Historic Interest
Wildlife

FACILITIES
Interpretive signs

In 2003, 144,000 acres burned in the park, and another 165,000 burned outside Glacier from several wildfires, including the 57,570-acre Roberts Fire, visible from this trail. All told, Northwest Montana fires covered more than 300,000 acres in 2003, a year when temperatures were among the hottest on record.

few white-ghost trees still stand—some burned-out trees remain erect for decades. These snags provide homes for a variety of bird species, including black-backed woodpeckers and northern hawk owls that nest in the cavities of dead trees. Most impressive is the new growth of primarily lodgepole pine, which depends on fire for regeneration. Lodgepoles produce serotinous cones, which open and release seeds only under extreme heat. Cones may await fire conditions for decades, finally regenerating a burned area with as many as 20,000 seedlings per acre in the newly open and sunny montane. The thick succession of seedlings is referred to as a dog-hair stand.

As the trail begins to climb and circle back, you will encounter numerous wildflowers, including fireweed, another colonizer of postfire areas. Part of the primrose family, the brilliant pink to magenta perennial grows 4-foot-tall spikes with many flowers per stalk. The seeds remain viable for years; after fire, they germinate in the newly open, sunny terrain.

Among the new growth are aspens; wild rose; a variety of grasses; and raspberry, strawberry, and thimbleberry. At the trail's highest point, look north for views of 9,000-foot peaks along the Continental Divide. You cross a small stream (do not drink the water) where a declining species, the boreal toad,

Wildflowers

Flora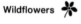

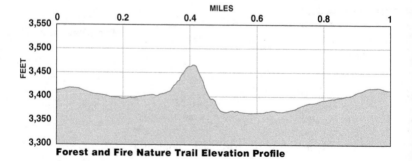

Forest and Fire Nature Trail Elevation Profile

Glacier Park Fire Firsts

NOTES

It was the first national park to have a fire crew and fire-management program. In the early 1920s, it was the first park to use the Canadian technology of portable horse-drawn water pumps to douse fire. Glacier was the first national park to build fire lookouts and, by 1923, had run phone lines to three lookouts. In 1946 Glacier became the first park to use smoke jumpers.

enjoys the shallows. Scientists are examining the effects of fire and UV radiation on the toads after a curious event: In the burn area following the Moose Fire, new breeding sites occurred, and park roads were closed while thousands of toadlets migrated across the pavement.

Wildlife

Water here flows into the North Fork of the Flathead River, which is visible as you look north. The river soon meets the Middle and South Forks

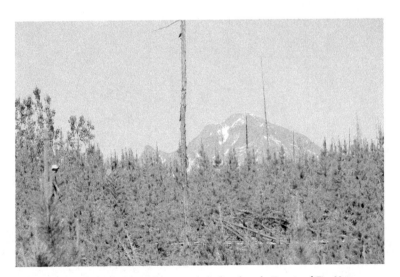

The cycle of burn and regrowth *is nature's display along the Forest and Fire Nature Trail, an area that burned in the 2001 Moose Fire.*

before flowing south into Flathead Lake, the largest natural freshwater lake in the west. Outbound Lower Flathead River is a tributary to the Columbia, which flows west to the Pacific Ocean.

MILESTONES

▶1	0.0	Start from just inside the park's Camas Creek entrance in the trail's parking area. The trailhead is on the northeast side of the paved parking area.
▶2	0.09	A trail sign directs walkers to continue south; the loop finishes here.
▶3	0.4	This is the highest point in elevation and a good place to view a forest in recovery.
▶4	0.9	The loop meets up with the trail.
▶5	1.0	Parking lot

Akokala Lake Trail

Akokala Lake Trail provides a gentle jaunt through a cedar, hemlock, and lodgepole pine zone, as well as wildfire-cleared meadows and scenic valleys. Hikers will enjoy excellent views of Numa Ridge Fire Lookout, Reuter Peak, and Mount Peabody, where few glimpses were visible a dozen years ago.

Best Time

The trail is among the early passable routes in spring—mostly snow-free by early June—and provides lovely fall colors well into October. Much of the trail is shady, so it can be a good choice on warm days.

Finding the Trail

From Bowman Lake, the trailhead begins at the north end of the campground loop. Park near the lake in the hikers' parking area, and walk north and counterclockwise on the campground vehicle loop to the trailhead, which is just after the top of the loop on the west side of the road. Note that the white wall tent, the official hospitality area, is open to visitors and provides up-to-date information on trail conditions, animal identification information, and a fire history display. Campground hosts can assist with any questions.

Trail Description

Initially, the trail ascends a low-elevation shoulder of Numa Ridge under a thick tree canopy. Here,

---

TRAIL USE
Day hiking, backpacking, youth-friendly

LENGTH
11.6 miles, 5–7 hours

VERTICAL FEET
±1,105'

DIFFICULTY
1 2 **3** 4 5

TRAIL TYPE
Out-and-back

SURFACE TYPE
Dirt and gravel

START & END
N48° 49.811'
W114° 12.277'

FEATURES
Lake
Fishing
Flora
Secluded
Geologic Interest
Historic Interest
Wildlife
Wildfire ecology
Views

FACILITIES
Ranger residence
Campground
Pit toilets
Potable water
Interpretive center
Backcountry campsites

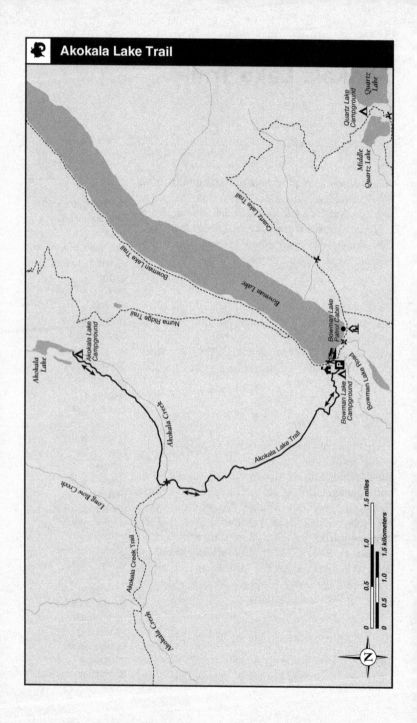

Akokala Lake Trail

Quartz Lake

Quartz Lake Campground

Middle Quartz Lake

Quartz Lake Trail

Bowman Lake Trail

Bowman Lake

Bowman Lake Patrol Cabin

Numa Ridge Trail

Akokala Lake Campground

Akokala Lake

Akokala Creek

Bowman Lake Campground

Bowman Lake Road

Akokala Lake Trail

Long Bow Creek

Akokala Creek Trail

Akokala Creek

0   0.5   1.0   1.5 miles

0   0.5   1.0   1.5 kilometers

N

the trail remains damp and cool nearly all summer, and in fact, a bog area guarantees mosquitoes for a few hundred yards. It's worth it because at 1.5 miles, the trees open up to bright wildflowers, such as beargrass and columbine. Look for huckleberries late July through September.

Flora

As you continue, listen for the rushing Akokala Creek as it tumbles west to meet the North Fork of the Flathead River just north of the Polebridge Ranger Station. Thanks to wildfires, such as the 2003 Wedge Canyon Fire, you can catch glimpses of several peaks ahead. Just after the log footbridge over Akokala Creek, at mile 3.47, the trail will come to a T and meet Akokala Creek Trail, which heads west and out of the park—stay right/east on Akokala Lake Trail heading through burned timber and grassy glades. Notice that the trail sign was scorched in the fires.

The Wedge Canyon Fire burned through here in 2003, scorching 30,300 acres inside the park and 53,400 acres outside Glacier.

The trail gently climbs alongside Akokala Creek, with several viewpoints of Numa Ridge to the southeast—look closely and you may pick out the Numa Ridge Fire Lookout, which sits at 6,960 feet elevation. To the left/north is 8,763-foot Reuter Peak, and straight ahead is 9,216-foot Mount Peabody.

Views

Summer's long days ripen the huckleberries, which attract both black and grizzly bears. You may notice strands of barbed wire fixed to trees on the

Wildlife

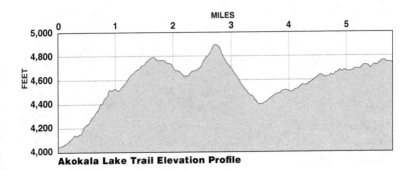

Akokala Lake Trail Elevation Profile

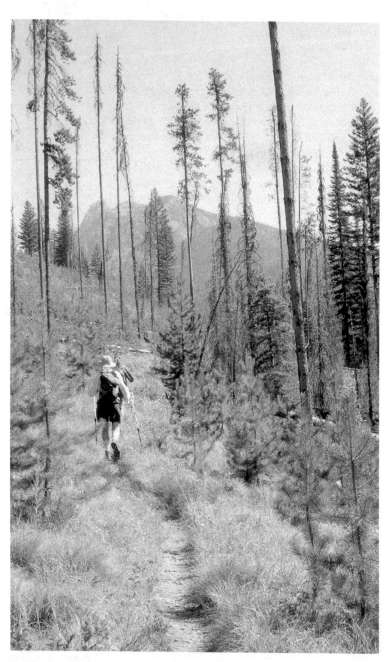

Akokala Lake Trail *is a study area for the Northern Divide Grizzly Bear Project.*

Akokala is the Kootenai Indian word for "place of red willows." Akokala had been the original name for Bowman Lake, notable for red willows at the head of Bowman Lake.

trail's south side. Researchers collect hair samples from these "rub trees" to determine the number of *Ursus americanus* (black bears) and *Ursus arctos horribilis* (grizzly bears). As always, make plenty of noise, carry bear-deterrent spray, and hike in groups.

The final 0.8 mile descends to the lake; the tree canopy becomes thick again. Look for Franklin grouse here as you spot shade-loving wildflowers. The campsite and pit toilet (a toilet bench with no walls) is just ahead on the right, near the stream's bank. Continue heading straight/north to the lake. There's not much room on the shore to picnic, but the views are worth the trip. The surrounding peaks seem to rise right out of the water. A bushwhacked trail scrambles around the narrow, half-mile-long, bottle-green lake, a route mostly used by moose and the occasional fisherman.

 Camping

 Lake

🚶 MILESTONES

►1	0.0	Start from Bowman Lake Campground.
►2	3.47	Bridge over Akokala Creek
►3	3.6	At T, take right/east trail.
►4	5.7	Spur trail to campsites and toilet
►5	5.8	Akokala Lake. Return to trailhead.

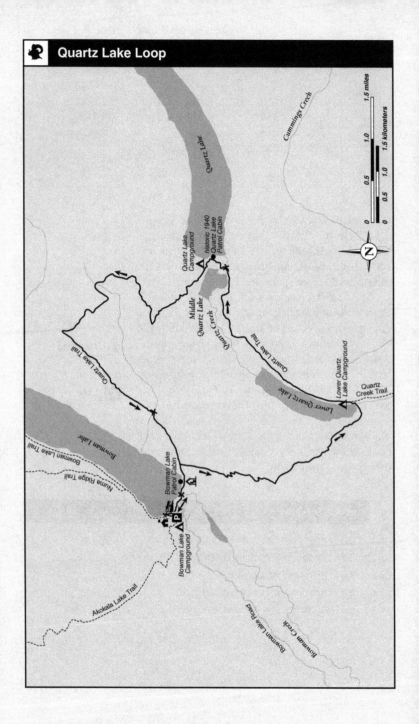

Quartz Lake Loop

Quartz Lake Loop

The Quartz Lake hike is a strenuous hike through a variety of forest ecosystems, but you're rewarded with views, huckleberries, a jump in the refreshing water, and loons. All three Quartz Lakes are nesting sites for common loons and, indeed, Glacier is home to about 20% of Montana's loon population. The seldom-viewed bird has a 3.5- to 4-foot wingspan and can weigh up to 12 pounds.

Best Time

The trail tends to remain damp or muddy on the north-facing side of Cerulean Ridge and drier and hotter on the south-facing Quartz Lakes side of the ridge but is generally snow-free by late June and accessible through early October.

Finding the Trail

From the Bowman Lake Boat Ramp at Bowman Lake Campground, find the large brown trailhead signs for both the Bowman Lake Trail, which sidles along the lake's north shore, and the Quartz Lake Trail, which initially follows Bowman Lake's south shore. The Quartz Lake Loop begins immediately right/south of the boat ramp; you'll see a small metal trail sign. Head east following the lake's shoreline, cross the large log footbridge over Bowman Creek, and hike on to the Quartz Lakes.

TRAIL USE
Day hiking, backpacking

LENGTH
12.9 miles, 5–7 hours

VERTICAL FEET
±1,490'

DIFFICULTY
1 2 **3 4** 5

TRAIL TYPE
Balloon

SURFACE TYPE
Dirt and gravel

START & END
N48° 49.746'
W114° 12.023'

FEATURES
Lakes
Fishing
Flora
Secluded
Geologic Interest
Historic Interest
Wildlife
Birds
Wildfire ecology

FACILITIES
Ranger residence
Campground
Pit toilets
Potable water
Interpretive center
Backcountry campsites

Look east to 9,638-
foot Vulture Peak.
One of the park's
remaining glaciers,
Vulture Glacier, is
tucked on the east
side. It's shrinking
at such a rate that
the U.S. Geological
Survey estimates it
will be gone by 2020.

Flora

Wildlife

Camping

Trail Description

After leaving the Bowman Lake area, the trail begins to climb Cerulean Ridge, where a trail sign sends hikers either to Lower Quartz Lake over Quartz Ridge or to Quartz Lake over Cerulean Ridge—either direction is a good choice for the loop; however, on hot days, consider departing early in the morning and heading counterclockwise toward Lower Quartz Lake first because this route has more switchbacks and is slightly steeper.

The gradual climb up Quartz Ridge is for huckleberry lovers. The route here on the Bowman Lake side of Quartz Ridge provides trailside bounty each August—remember that bears and other animals and birds need to share that bounty. Park regulations allow you to pick only what you can eat and to take no more than one quart of huckleberries per person per day. Make lots of noise through the tall timbers to avoid surprising wildlife.

As you pop over the ridgetop at 5,082 feet elevation, you see the Logging Ridge ahead. Sometimes the trail has brief washouts from spring runoff—a hiking pole is handy. Once at Lower Quartz Lake, 4,240 feet elevation, you'll cross a footbridge over Quartz Creek and find a small campground with pit toilets. Note that Quartz Creek Trail, a horsemen's favorite, splits off here, heading directly south 7 miles to the Inside

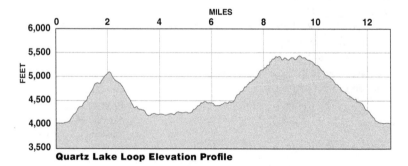

Quartz Lake Loop Elevation Profile

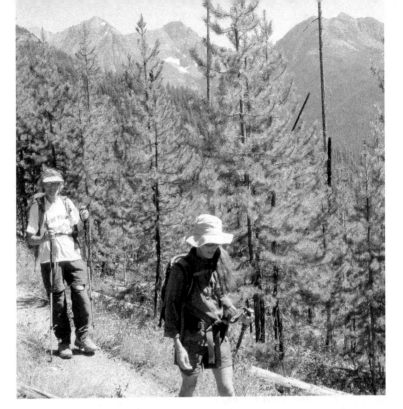

Hikers along *the Quartz Lake Loop.*

North Fork Road (which is only seasonally open to vehicles). Stay on the Quartz Lake Loop by hiking north and along Lower Quartz Lake. Listen for loons.

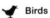 Birds

The trail cruises above the lakeshore, into the woods again to Middle Quartz Lake at 4,397 feet elevation. It's just a couple of minutes more to Quartz Lake, one of the park's larger backcountry lakes at 4 miles long and 0.5 mile wide. The historic 1940 Quartz Lake Patrol Cabin and its picturesque pebble beach provide a lovely photo subject and picnic spot, although the campground is just another 0.1 mile ahead.

 Lake

The trail ascends Cerulean Ridge, climbing among new growth and patches of trees that survived the 1988 Red Bench Fire, providing views of

 Historic Interest

Loons frequent the lakes of Northwest Montana, and you may hear their lonely call before you see the reclusive birds. They are not ducks but instead belong to the Gaviidae family—distant relatives to penguins and albatross—and therefore have dense bone structure, necessitating a long takeoff paddle to gain flight. If you hear loons, approach the lake quietly, and they may continue their woeful call.

Logging Mountain and Vulture Peak, where Vulture Glacier hangs just out of sight. At 5,380 feet, the trail **Summit** ▲ summit, it's a downhill shady cruise to Bowman Lake with few views—but more huckleberries!

🚶 MILESTONES

►1	0.0	Start from Bowman Lake Boat Ramp.
►2	0.18	Cross Bowman Creek.
►3	0.35	See the patrol cabin on the lake side of the trail.
►4	0.58	Trail sign at T indicates right/south to Lower Quartz Lake or left/northeast to Upper Quartz Lake; both directions involve ascents and descents.
►5	3.62	Lower Quartz Lake and cross Quartz Creek.
►6	6.15	Middle Quartz Lake
►7	6.35	Cross Quartz Lake inlet.
►8	6.54	Quartz Lake and the historic 1940 Quartz Lake Patrol Cabin
►9	12.3	Keep straight at trail junction.
►10	12.9	Bowman Lake Boat Ramp

Logging Lake Trail

Logging Lake Trail used to be a ho-hum hike until a few wildfires opened up the tree canopy, providing superb views of Glacier's seldom-seen Logging Creek region. Logging Lake Trail is an excellent choice for novice hikers and backpackers because the 5.5 miles to the foot of the lake covers gentle terrain, provides limited forest protection from sun or weather, and offers a variety of views. While this hike is decorated with wildflowers, such as trillium, sticky geranium, and Indian paintbrush, few huckleberry bushes line the trail—a surprise since huckleberries are prolific in nearby drainages. There are, however, lots of thimbleberries and occasionally nettles.

Best Time

The trail can be accessed when the road opens in early June through October, if you don't mind mud and patches of snow in shady sections. Some sections remain damp into early August.

Finding the Trail

Driving from Polebridge Ranger Station, immediately turn right/south at the T following the Inside North Fork Road (Glacier Route 7), 7 miles to the trailhead at Logging Creek. This seasonal gravel road is rough and narrow. The trailhead is immediately before a bridge over Logging Creek—you've gone too far if you see the ranger's residence on the right/west and Logging Campground on the left/

TRAIL USE
Day hiking, backpacking, child-friendly
LENGTH
11.0 miles, 4–6 hours
VERTICAL FEET
±471'
DIFFICULTY
1 **2** 3 4 5
TRAIL TYPE
Out-and-back
SURFACE TYPE
Dirt and gravel
START & END
N48° 41.949'
W114° 11.617'

FEATURES
Lake
Flora
Secluded
Geologic Interest
Historic Interest
Wildlife
Birds

FACILITIES
Ranger station
Lodging
Restaurants
Store
Gas
Campgrounds

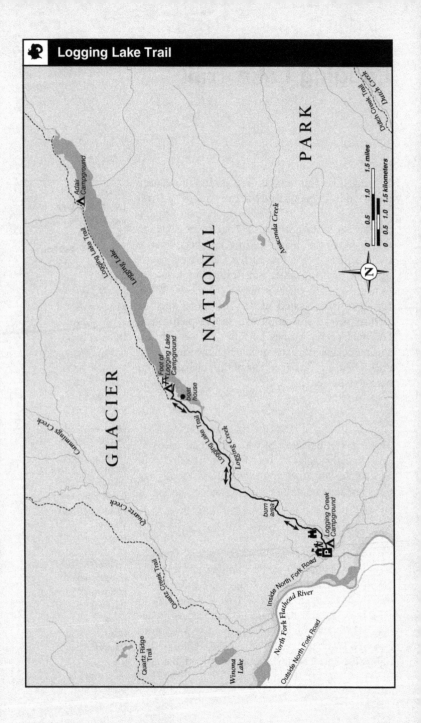

east. Park at the pullout north of the bridge, and see the trail signs on the left/east side of the road.

Trail Description

The route follows Logging Creek up to the lake, although sometimes the trail is high on a bench away from the foamy stream. Here, you experience solitude and silence, perhaps punctuated by the sounds of the pileated woodpecker, Steller's jay, and black-capped chickadee. You may also find old, partially burned communication wires from an era past.

 Secluded

 Birds

 Flora

 Wildlife

As the trail wends in and out of new and old growth hemlock, lodgepole pine, and occasional ponderosa pine forest, hikers encounter wetlands and shallow creek crossings. The damp mud provides an imprinted tale of travelers: deer, black bear, moose, human, horse, and pack mule—and mosquitoes in early summer.

The first glimpse of 5-mile-long Logging Lake is that of emerald waters surrounded by thick forest and backdropped by Adair Ridge on the lake's south shore, the 8,375-foot Mount Geduhn to the east, and Logging Ridge to the north. It's another few trail minutes to the junction down to the beach, lake, and campsites. The lake is shallow quite a ways out, perfect for wading and swimming. Fly-fishing

 Lake

 Camping

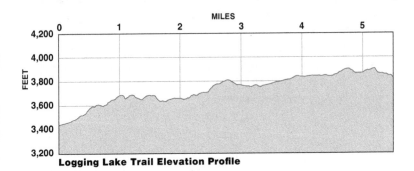

Logging Lake Trail Elevation Profile

The Kootenai Indians called the lake Big Beaver Lake after a tale of a 20-foot-long beaver residing there; however, Logging Lake, Creek, and Mountain are so named for significant logging of ponderosa pines in the 1890s, some three decades before Glacier became a national park.

A watering can at the campsite's picnic area encourages visitors to water seedlings planted as part of Glacier's native-plant restoration program, begun in the 1970s to revegetate backcountry campgrounds and remove exotic plants.

is tricky unless you don't mind wading or you pack an inflatable craft. The rewards are many: Large bull trout and lake trout troll the deeper portions of the lake, while whitefish and small trout seek midges in shallow areas. Note that the eastern/upper portion of Logging Lake is closed to fishing because of nesting bald eagles.

From the campsite junction, the Logging Lake Patrol Cabin is another 0.25 mile east. Beyond and farther eastward is the Adair Campground at 2.6 additional miles and Grace Lake another 4.6 miles from the foot of Logging Lake Campground.

🚶 MILESTONES

▶1 0.0   Start from Inside North Fork Road at Logging Creek bridge.
▶2 0.5   Fires cleared timber, allowing views of several peaks.
▶3 1.4   Burn area
▶4 4.5   See Logging Lake.
▶5 5.15 Junction; take right trail to pit toilets, campsites, picnic area, beach, and lake.
▶6 5.5   Logging Lake. Return to trailhead.

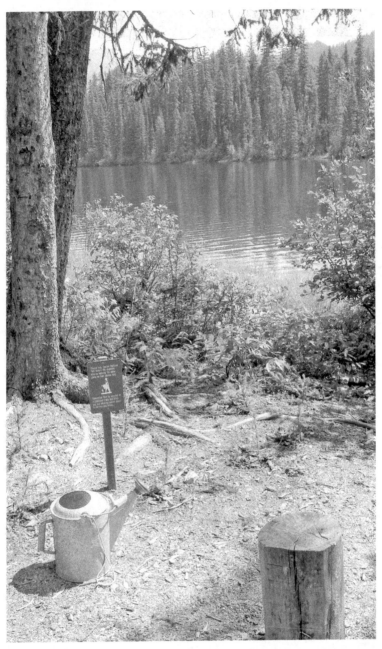

An effort to revegetate *impacted backcountry campsites encourages watering-can assistance from hikers at Logging Lake.*

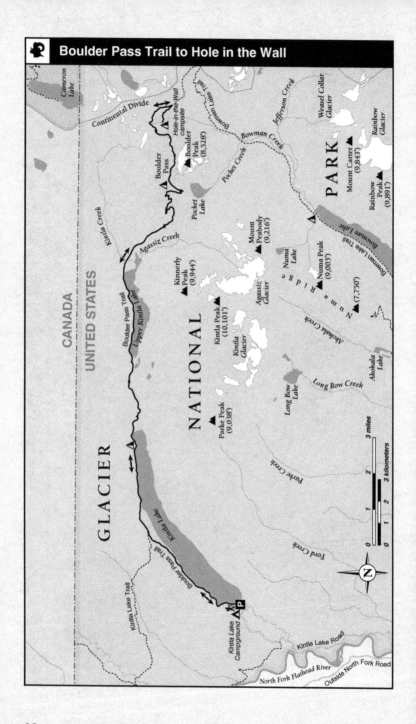

Cameron Lake

Continental Divide

Bowman Lake Trail

Jefferson Creek

Weasel Collar Glacier

Rainbow Glacier

Hole-in-the-Wall campsite

Boulder Pass

Boulder Peak (8,528')

Bowman Creek

P A R K

Mount Carter (9,843')

Kintla Creek

Pocket Creek

Pocket Lake

Rainbow Peak (9,891')

Agassiz Creek

Mount Peabody (9,216')

Bowman Lake Trail

Bowman Lake

CANADA

UNITED STATES

Kinnerly Peak (9,944')

Agassiz Glacier

Numa Lake

Numa Peak (9,003')

(7,750')

N u m a   R i d g e

Boulder Pass Trail

Upper Kintla Lake

Kintla Peak (10,101')

Kintla Glacier

Akokala Creek

Akokala Lake

N A T I O N A L

Long Bow Creek

Long Bow Lake

Parke Peak (9,038')

G L A C I E R

Kintla Lake

Parke Creek

3 miles

3 kilometers

Kintla Lake Trail

Ford Creek

Boulder Pass Trail

Z

Kintla Lake Campground

P

Kintla Lake Road

North Fork Flathead River

Outside North Fork Road

Boulder Pass Trail to Hole in the Wall

Thick timber forest cruising begins the hike to one of Glacier's most spectacular backcountry spots: Hole in the Wall. The first campground at the head of Kintla Lake features a strange contraption called a precipitator, left over from the failed 1901 Butte Oil Well. The next campgrounds, at Upper Kintla Lake and Boulder Pass, provide exceedingly fewer bugs and more mountain views. The apex of scenes and campsites is in the Hole in the Wall cirque, which features a dozen waterfalls, thousands of wildflowers, and a resident grizzly bear sow and cub of the year. To finish this horseshoe-shaped, five-day trip, travelers continue down a different drainage to another shoreline hike along Bowman Lake and exit at Bowman Campground.

Best Time

The trail is fully accessible early August through late September, although you should check with the rangers regarding several snow/ice crossings in and near Boulder Pass. Also, check for trail or campsite closures due to bear activity.

Finding the Trail

This discussion begins at Kintla Lake Campground, 14.3 miles north of Polebridge, where the trail climbs through two passes, ending at Bowman Lake, although the route could be hiked in the reverse. Boulder Pass Trailhead is 0.1 mile before Kintla Lake Campground, on the left/north side of Kintla Road; a spur to the trail begins in the

TRAIL USE
Backpacking

LENGTH
40.0 miles or 33.4-mile horseshoe, 4–6 days

VERTICAL FEET
+12,032'/-12,049'

DIFFICULTY
1 2 3 4 **5**

TRAIL TYPE
Out-and-back or horseshoe with shuttle

SURFACE TYPE
Dirt, gravel, rock, snow, and ice

START
N48° 56.118'
W114° 20.947'

END
BOWMAN LAKE TRAILHEAD:
N48° 49.760'
W114° 12.020'

FEATURES
Flora
Geologic Interest
Historic Interest
Wildlife
Lakes, Fishing
Waterfalls, Views

FACILITIES
Ranger station
Pit toilet
Potable water
Campgrounds

Lake

Flora

Views

northeast portion of Kintla Lake Campground at site 12, close to the lake.

To make this hike a 33.4-mile horseshoe, leave a shuttle vehicle at Bowman Lake's backcountry hikers' parking area. Some hikers leave a vehicle at Bowman Lake and then mountain bike 18 miles back to Kintla Lake.

Trail Description

The walk along the northwest shoreline of the 4.9-mile-long by 0.9-mile-wide Kintla Lake provides views of Parke Ridge to the south of the rolling trek. The southern shore was burned in the 2003 Wedge Canyon Fire, one of three major fires that summer that blazed through 144,000 acres in Glacier. Between Kintla and Upper Kintla Lakes, hikers are treated to glimpses of 10,101-foot Kintla Peak. It's ultimately 10.9 miles to Upper Kintla Campground on a trail replete with brushy sections of thick cow parsnip and thimbleberry.

A 3,250-foot climb begins at Upper Kintla, which sits only 2 miles from the Canadian border over the Boundary Mountains. Excellent views of Agassiz Glacier might keep your mind off the grueling switchbacks. Named after the father of

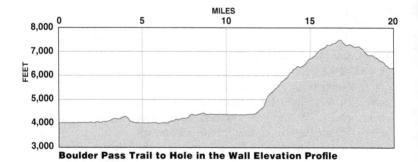

Boulder Pass Trail to Hole in the Wall Elevation Profile

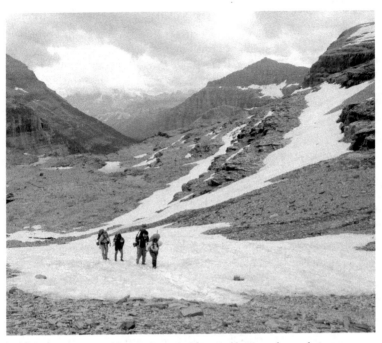

By early August, *most of the snow has melted from Boulder Pass, where a glacier once encased the area.*

glaciology, Louis Agassiz, this glacier is a shrinking 250 acres in a cirque under Kintla Peak.

Boulder Pass Campground sits below and west of the pass in a hanging valley that lives up to its name: Boulder Valley. Icy ponds, grass, and occasional summer snowstorms surround the three tent sites and food-prep area.

Camping

Above the treeline, the trail climbs to Boulder Pass and provides new views every few steps. The pass is a hanging valley with several ponds and many marmots. Cairns mark the trail through the snow. Some snow patches are quite steep, making hiking poles necessary. Some hikers use crampons here if conditions are icy. Once through Boulder

Pass, the 1,170-foot descent is on the youngest rock of the Belt series, red rock of the Kintla Formation. Hole in the Wall cirque, surrounded by Mount Custer and Boulder Peak, opens up ahead as the trail follows the ridge wall—there is some exposure, as well as steep snow crossings. Yellow columbine, Indian paintbrush, and mountain forget-me-nots line the trail. Hole in the Wall Campground sits between streams; the food-prep area is next to a mini waterfall and is perfect for filtering water. The campground also has the park's nicest composting toilet—large enough to change clothes inside. Plan to stay at Hole in the Wall a few nights to explore the talus slopes, see wildlife, and notice the oldest exposed rock, the billion-year-old stromatolites in the Helena limestone near the top of Hole in the Wall Falls. Across the next valley, Thunderbird Mountain and Weasel Collar Glacier are prominent.

Because Hole in the Wall campsites are very popular, you should secure reservations months in advance, but walk-ins to the Backcountry Offices may have a chance to acquire last-minute sites. If continuing down to Bowman Lake, note that there is a challenging cliff-edge stream crossing with lots of exposure. Brown Pass Campground's water source is 0.2 mile west of the campground. (See Trail 15: Bowman Lake Trail to Goat Haunt for the full trail description.)

Wildflowers

Waterfall

Geologic Interest

Hole in the Wall is
named for a hole in
the ground where the
stream disappears. It
reappears as a falls.

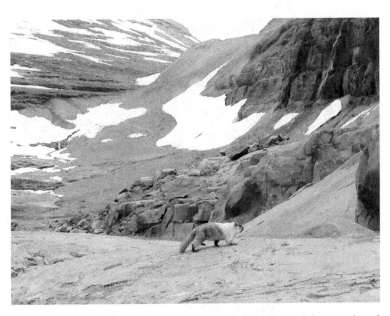

Hoary marmots, *named for the silvery guard hairs on their shoulders and chest, own the real estate in the Boulder Pass area.*

🚶 **MILESTONES**

▶1	0.0	Start from Kintla Lake Campground at the Boulder Pass Trailhead.
▶2	3.46	Junction with Kintla Trail/Starvation Creek; stay right/east
▶3	5.8	Head of Kintla Lake; campsite and patrol cabin
▶4	8.6	Upper Kintla Lake
▶5	10.9	Upper Kintla Lake Campground
▶6	11.3	Cross Kintla Creek.
▶7	16.0	Boulder Pass
▶8	18.9	Junction with Hole in the Wall Campsite Trail
▶9	20.0	Hole in the Wall Campsite

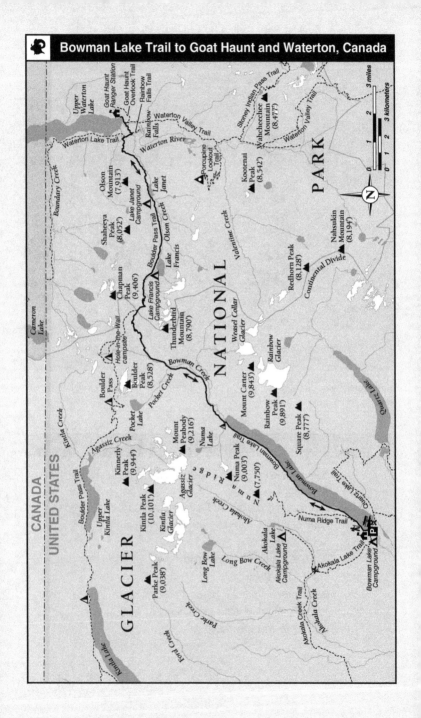

Bowman Lake Trail to Goat Haunt and Waterton, Canada

Upper Waterton Lake

Goat Haunt Ranger Station

Goat Haunt Overlook Trail

Rainbow Falls Trail

Waterton Valley Trail

Waterton Lake Trail

Waterton River

Rainbow Falls

Stoney Indian Pass Trail

Wahcheechee Mountain (8,477')

Waterton Valley Trail

Porcupine Lookout Trail

Olson Mountain (7,913')

Lake Janet

Kootenai Peak (8,542')

PARK

Lake Janet Campground

Olson Creek

Shaheeya Peak (8,052')

Boulder Pass Trail

Lake Francis

Nahsukin Mountain (8,194')

Chapman Peak (9,406')

Lake Francis Campground

Redhorn Peak (8,128')

Continental Divide

Cameron Lake

Hole-in-the-Wall campsite

Thunderbird Mountain (8,790')

NATIONAL

Weasel Collar Glacier

Valentine Creek

Boulder Pass

Boulder Peak (8,528')

Bowman Creek

Rainbow Glacier

Boundary Creek

Pocket Creek

Mount Carter (9,843')

Pocket Lake

Rainbow Peak (9,891')

Square Peak (8,777)

Kintla Creek

Agassiz Creek

Mount Peabody (9,216)

Numa Lake

Kinnerly Peak (9,944')

Numa Ridge

Bowman Lake Trail

Quartz Lake

CANADA

UNITED STATES

Boulder Pass Trail

Upper Kintla Lake

Kintla Peak (10,101')

Kintla Glacier

Agassiz Glacier

Numa Peak (9,003)

Akokala Creek

Bowman Lake

Quartz Lake Trail

Numa Ridge Trail

GLACIER

Parke Peak (9,038')

Long Bow Lake

Long Bow Creek

Akokala Lake

Akokala Lake Campground

Bowman Lake Campground

Akokala Lake Trail

Ford Creek

Kintla Lake

Parke Creek

Akokala Creek Trail

Akokala Creek

Bowman Lake Trail to Goat Haunt and Waterton, Canada

Not only does this trail cross the Continental Divide, it also crosses the international boundary between the United States and Canada. This hike begins on the west side of the divide among thick forests and climbs steeply to Brown Pass, where the vegetation gives way to views of glaciers, dramatic peaks, and waterfalls. Eastward from Brown Pass, the floral show provides trailside bouquets as the route eases downward past lakes, campsites, and, finally, the head of Waterton Lake at Goat Haunt Ranger Station. A valid passport is required to enter Canada.

Best Time

The trail is snow-free late July through October, but the tour boat, the *MV International,* only operates mid-June through early September. Check locally regarding stream crossings, snow crossings, and trail closures due to bear activity.

Finding the Trail

At Bowman Lake Campground (6.3 miles northeast of Polebridge), park near the picnic area and walk through the campground. The Bowman Lake Trailhead is between campsites 16 and 18. You can also access the Bowman Lake Trailhead from the Bowman Lake boat ramp by walking north on the beach and past the dock to the trailhead signs.

TRAIL USE
Backpacking
LENGTH
22.3 miles, 3–6 days
VERTICAL FEET
+8,347'/-8,143'
DIFFICULTY
1 2 3 4 **5**
TRAIL TYPE
Point-to-point
SURFACE TYPE
Dirt, gravel, rock, snow, and lake shuttle boat
START
N48° 49.755'
W114° 12.045'
END
N48° 57.571'
W113° 53.306'

FEATURES
Flora
Secluded
Geologic Interest
Historic Interest
Wildlife
Birds
Lakes
Waterfalls

FACILITIES
Ranger station
Interpretive center tent
Campgrounds
Pit toilets

Trait Description

Lake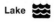

Wildlife

Flora

Birds

Camping ⚠

The Bowman Lake Trail parallels the lake's north shore, although few access points slip down to the water; instead, the trail rolls among thick dog-haired lodgepole pine, Douglas fir, and Devil's Club. Whitetail deer, mountain lions, and bears like the shade and food sources here: thimbleberries, shade-loving Oregon grapes, and striped coralroot. The lake hosts loons, osprey, and bald eagles.

The Head of Bowman Lake Campground offers flat tent sites, a food-prep area with a fire pit, and pit toilets. This is also where canoes are stashed and paddlers begin the long climb to Brown Pass. Thimbleberry bushes clog the trail and, in some places, completely hide the footpath. The trail crosses a dry creek bed where you can see the upcoming climb to the northeast. Then it's back into the woods among 6-foot-tall cow parsnip and thimbleberries nearly all the way to Brown Pass Campground. The final mile switchbacks and stair-steps up the pass—watch for stinging nettles. The campground is at the base of a massive 2011 avalanche that cleared trees from Chapman Peak. It's very buggy here—bring mosquito head netting and bug repellent!

One option for fit backpackers is to skip Brown Pass and camp another 2.1 miles up the trail at Hole

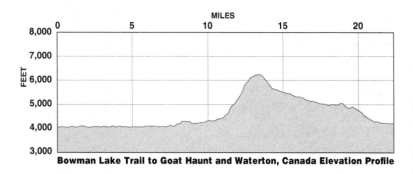

Bowman Lake Trail to Goat Haunt and Waterton, Canada Elevation Profile

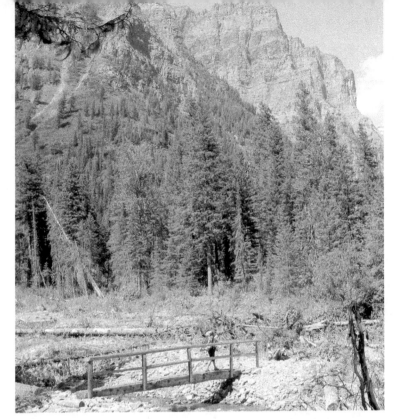

Bowman Lake Trail, *between upper Bowman Lake and the stair-step climb to the pass, crosses several streambeds.*

in the Wall Campground (see Trail 14 for details). Between Brown Pass and Hole in the Wall, look westward for an astonishing view of Bowman Lake. Even if you don't camp at Hole in the Wall, it's worth the extra climb before retracing your steps back to Brown Pass, the Continental Divide, and cruising eastward and down to Hawksbill, Lake Francis, or Lake Janet Campgrounds. Just below the last switchback, at the astonishingly brilliant turquoise Thunderbird Pond, look up at Thunderbird Falls gushing from Thunderbird Glacier on Thunderbird Mountain.

 Waterfall

From Lake Francis, Dixon Glacier is visible above the trail and under a knob called The Sentinel. The remainder of the trail cruises between peaks, such

Goat Haunt Ranger Station is named for Goat Haunt Lake and Mountain, where the white goats scamper.

as Citadel to the south and Olson Mountain to the north. Streamlets nurture monkey flower, penstemon, and columbine. At the final junction, turn right/south for Goat Haunt Port of Entry, the boat dock and the *MV International* tour boat, Goat Haunt Shelter Cabins, and Waterton River Campground. A left/north turn takes you on the 8-mile Waterton Lake Trail that crosses into Canada at Boundary Bay—and the route if you miss the tour boat!

🚶 MILESTONES

▶1	0.0	Bowman Lake Campground
▶2	0.75	Junction with Numa Lookout Trail; continue eastward.
▶3	7.1	Head of Bowman Lake Campground
▶4	13.55	Water source for Brown Pass Campground
▶5	13.75	Brown Pass Campground
▶6	13.90	Brown Pass and junction with Boulder Pass/Hole in the Wall
▶7	16.0	Hawksbill Campground
▶8	16.25	Junction with spur trail to Lake Francis Campground
▶9	19.0	Lake Janet Campground
▶10	22.0	Junction with Waterton Lake Trail; stay right/south for Goat Haunt Ranger Station, shelter, and boat dock.
▶11	22.1	Junction with Rainbow Fall Trail; stay left for Goat Haunt.
▶12	22.2	Hanging bridge over the Waterton River
▶13	22.3	Goat Haunt Ranger Station, shelter, and boat dock

NOTES

At 5,525 miles, the international boundary between Glacier and Waterton is part of the longest undefended border between the U.S. and Canada. Because of rugged, mountainous terrain, surveyors in the 1870s installed markers and cleared a 20-foot swath through the woods and across the mountains.

Backpackers might consider a rendezvous with other back-packers to exchange car keys midway through the trail, with one group hiking from Bowman Lake and the other group from Waterton/Goat Haunt, and riding the *MV International* tour boat on Waterton Lake. Another delightful shortcut is to canoe or motorboat (motorized vehicles are limited to 10 horsepower or less) the length of Bowman Lake to avoid the 6.7-mile shoreline hike.

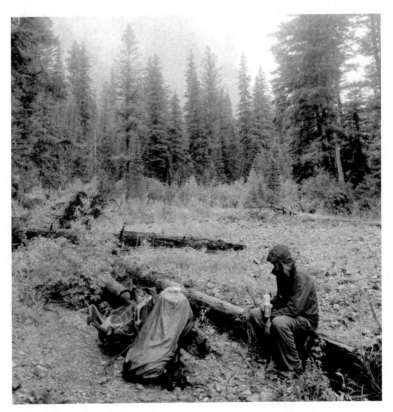

Brown Pass Campground's *food-prep area affords views of a massive avalanche path that scrubbed trees from the pass area.*

CHAPTER 2

Logan Pass and Saint Mary Area

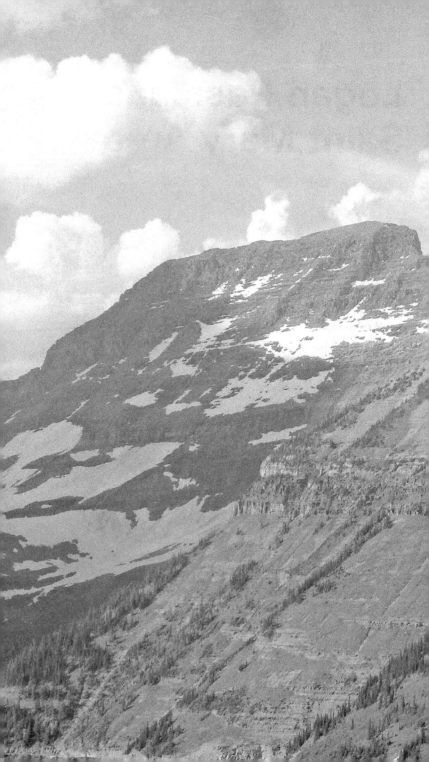

Logan Pass and Saint Mary Area

Climate zones collide at Logan Pass, where the Pacific Maritime weather of the West Side meets the Prairie/Arctic temperatures and vegetation of the east side of the Continental Divide, creating a visible and stark contrast in foliage and landscape. Snowed in for much of the year, Logan Pass, at 6,647 feet in elevation, often has plenty of snow, even in July, for tossing snowballs and tromping in the summer slush. Several popular hiking trails depart from Logan Pass and from trailheads a few miles below the pass along Going-to-the Sun Road. These trails access the high alpine that cloisters many of the park's remaining glaciers. It's here that visitors can get a good look at the glaciation that occurred when ice sheets retreated as recently as 10,000 to 12,000 years ago at the end of the most recent ice age. It's also here in the high country that visitors are most likely to see Glacier's iconic mountain goats as they climb the rocks or graze at roadside. While mountain goats (*Oreamnos americanus*) seem curious and may approach people, it is not safe to be in close proximity to the horned goats; indeed, park regulations forbid people from being closer than 25 yards from the park's white goats and other ungulates (hooved mammals). Park rangers advise visitors to stay at least 100 yards away from bears and wolves for everyone's safety.

Only the Saint Mary Campground remains open year-round, but few services are available in winter, plus the Saint Mary Campground is on primitive status and does not have flush toilets or potable water from December 1 to March 31. A few commercial or forest service campgrounds outside the park boundary in and near the gateway community of Saint Mary are open most of the year. Rising Sun Campground and its neighboring cabins, café, camp store, and boat dock (open summers only) provide a lovely launch for daytime activities.

Opposite and overleaf: *The Garden Wall, a glacial arête leading northward from Logan Pass, is the Continental Divide and hosts the Highline Trail, aka the Continental Divide Trail.*

Logan Pass and Saint Mary Area

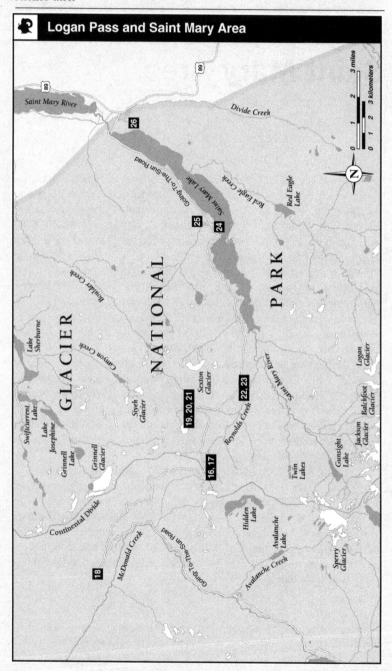

TRAIL FEATURES TABLE

Logan Pass and Saint Mary Area

TRAIL	DIFFICULTY	LENGTH	TYPE	USES & ACCESS	TERRAIN	FLORA & FAUNA	OTHER
16	2	5.14	Out-and-back	Day Hiking, Child-Friendly	Lake	Flora, Wildlife	Geologic Interest, Historic Interest
17	2–3	15.2	Out-and-back	Day Hiking, Child-Friendly		Flora, Wildlife	Secluded, Views, Geologic Interest, Historic Interest
18	4	8.4	Out-and-back	Day Hiking, Child-Friendly		Flora, Wildfire Ecology	Secluded, Views, Photo Opportunity, Geologic Interest, Historic Interest
19	2	2.5	Point-to-point	Day Hiking, Child-Friendly		Flora, Birds, Wildlife	Secluded, Views, Geologic Interest, Historic Interest
20	4–5	10.3	Point-to-point	Day Hiking		Flora, Birds, Wildlife	Secluded, Views, Geologic Interest, Historic Interest
21	3	9.0	Out-and-back	Day Hiking	Glacier	Flora, Wildlife	Secluded, Geologic Interest, Historic Interest
22	3–4	12.6	Out-and-back	Day Hiking, Backpacking	Lake, Waterfall, Glacier	Flora, Wildlife	Secluded, Fishing, Geologic Interest, Historic Interest
23	2–3	4.5	Point-to-point	Day Hiking, Child-Friendly	Lake, Waterfall	Flora, Birds, Wildlife	Secluded, Geologic Interest, Historic Interest
24	2	5.0	Out-and-back	Day Hiking, Child-Friendly	Waterfall	Flora, Wildlife	Secluded, Geologic Interest
25	3	10.5	Out-and-back	Day Hiking, Child-Friendly	Lake	Flora, Birds, Wildlife	Secluded, Fishing, Views, Photo Opportunity, Geologic Interest, Historic Interest
26	1	3.5	Loop	Day Hiking, Child-Friendly		Flora, Birds, Wildlife	Secluded, Geologic Interest, Historic Interest

Legend

USES & ACCESS
- Day Hiking
- Backpacking
- Horses
- Child-Friendly
- Ski/Snowshoe
- Wheelchair Access

TYPE
- Loop
- Balloon
- Out-and-back
- Point-to-point

DIFFICULTY
- 1 2 3 4 5 +
less   more

TERRAIN
- Lake
- Waterfall
- Glacier

FLORA & FAUNA
- Flora
- Birds
- Wildlife
- Wildfire Ecology

OTHER
- Secluded
- Swimming
- Fishing
- Views
- Photo Opportunity
- Geologic Interest
- Historic Interest

Permits and Maps

A fishing permit is not required to fish in Glacier, but a Montana fishing license is required outside the park, and a Conservation/Recreation Use Permit is required for all activities on the Blackfeet Reservation (call 406-338-7207 for information). Fishing is catch-and-release only in certain areas for cutthroat trout—check with the entrance stations or ranger stations for details. The daily catch-and-possession limit is five fish, with a maximum of two cutthroat trout, two burbot (ling), one northern pike, two mountain whitefish, five lake whitefish, five kokanee salmon, five grayling, five rainbow trout, and five lake trout. The following creeks are closed to fishing for their entire length: Ole, Park, Muir, Coal, Nyack, Fish, Lee, Otatso, Boulder, and Kennedy Creeks.

Free park maps are available at entrance stations. Each of the park's lodging properties offers rudimentary local-area maps with details of trailhead access. Excellent maps are available for purchase at the in-park bookstores, gift shops, and grocery stores, as well as through the Glacier National Park Conservancy's bookstore in the West Glacier train depot, sporting goods shops, and general stores outside the park and online.

Opposite: *Virginia Falls feeds a series of waterfalls that splash into the St. Mary River, and is one of the most popular family hikes in Glacier.*

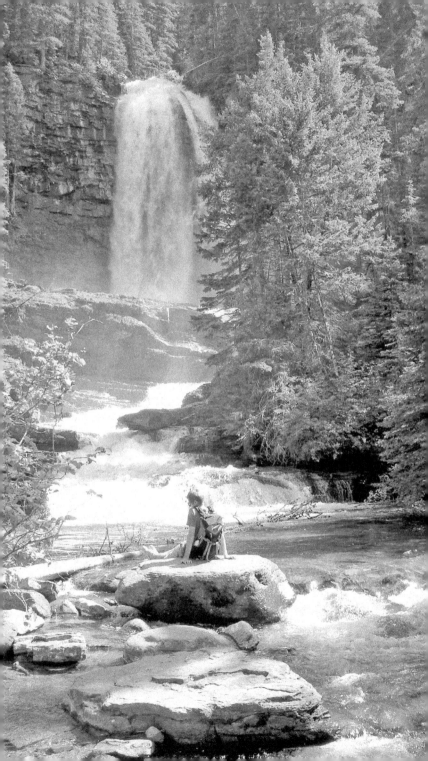

Logan Pass and Saint Mary Area

Siyeh Bend Trail and Piegan Pass Trail (Siyeh Bend to Jackson Glacier Overlook) 137

On the east side of Logan Pass, the Siyeh Bend Trail connects to the Piegan Pass Trail for an easy half-loop route that is below the snow line by late spring, when Going-to-the-Sun Road may not be completely open to Logan Pass. This trip is perfect for hikers who are itching to get into the backcountry.

TRAIL 19

Day hiking, child-friendly
2.5 miles
Point-to-point
Difficulty 1 **2** 3 4 5

Siyeh Pass Trail (Siyeh Bend to Sunrift Gorge) 143

One of Glacier's premier trails is an all-day backcountry trek that cruises through wildflower meadows and pine and spruce forests, with views of glaciers. The route travels near the terminal moraine of Sexton Glacier at the park's highest-elevation pass at 8,080 feet before descending past glacial tarns and waterfalls and ending along the scoured-smooth red argillite walls of Sunrift Gorge, and the shuttle back to your vehicle.

TRAIL 20

Day hiking
10.3 miles
Point-to-point
Difficulty 1 2 3 **4 5**

Piegan Pass Trail 147

Much of the Piegan Pass Trail is visible to hikers from the trailhead, as they look upward and to the north and east where the trail climbs above treeline, crosses snow patches as late as the end of July, and provides views of three glaciers: Blackfoot, Jackson, and the trail's namesake, Piegan Glacier, as hikers summit the pass. The next scene is down into the Many Glacier area, yet another spectacular view and an additional 12.85 miles on to Many Glacier Lodge.

TRAIL 21

Day hiking
9.0 miles
Out-and-back
Difficulty 1 2 **3** 4 5

Otokomi Lake/Rose Creek Trail..... 167

This gentle climb from the Rising Sun Camp Store cruises between Otokomi Mountain and Goat Mountain, often over July snow patches, before reaching the trout-thick Otokomi Lake and campsites, an area known for its popularity with the grizzly bear community. The trail is sometimes closed due to bear activity, so check with rangers before making hiking plans.

TRAIL 25

Day hiking,
youth-friendly
10.5 miles
Out-and-back
Difficulty 1 2 **3** 4 5

Beaver Pond Trail................. 173

An excellent choice for new and young hikers, the Beaver Pond Trail easily rolls through two distinct scenes: a thick aspen and pine forest to the ponds and open prairie meadows with views of Saint Mary Lake and surrounding peaks, plus the Historic 1913 Ranger Station at the trailhead.

TRAIL 26

Day hiking,
child-friendly
3.5 miles
Loop
Difficulty **1** 2 3 4 5

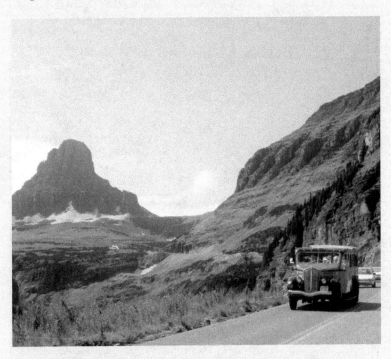

Glacier's fleet *of 33 historic, restored 1930s Red "Jammer" Buses transport guests across Going-to-the-Sun Road, and are so named for the drivers' jamming of the gears.*

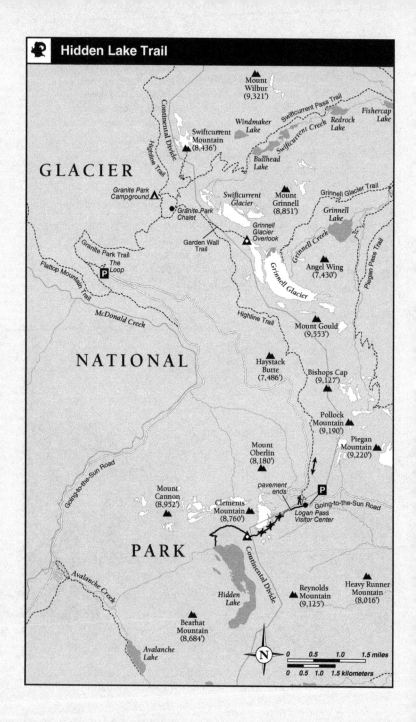

GLACIER

NATIONAL

PARK

Mount
Wilbur
(9,321')

Windmaker
Lake

Swiftcurrent Pass Trail

Swiftcurrent
Mountain
(8,436')

Redrock
Lake

Fishercap
Lake

Swiftcurrent Creek

Bullhead
Lake

Continental Divide

Highline Trail

Granite Park
Campground

Granite Park
Chalet

Swiftcurrent
Glacier

Mount
Grinnell
(8,851')

Grinnell Glacier Trail

Grinnell
Lake

Grinnell
Glacier
Overlook

Garden Wall
Trail

Grinnell Creek

Angel Wing
(7,430')

Piegan Pass Trail

Granite Park Trail

The
Loop

Flattop Mountain Trail

McDonald Creek

Grinnell Glacier

Highline Trail

Mount Gould
(9,553')

Haystack
Butte
(7,486')

Bishops Cap
(9,127')

Pollock
Mountain
(9,190')

Piegan
Mountain
(9,220')

Mount
Oberlin
(8,180')

pavement
ends

Going-to-the-Sun Road

Mount
Cannon
(8,952')

Clements
Mountain
(8,760')

Logan Pass
Visitor Center

Going-to-the-Sun Road

Continental Divide

Hidden
Lake

Reynolds
Mountain
(9,125')

Heavy Runner
Mountain
(8,016')

Avalanche Creek

Bearhat
Mountain
(8,684')

Avalanche
Lake

N

0   0.5   1.0   1.5 miles

0   0.5   1.0   1.5 kilometers

Hidden Lake Trail

The Hidden Lake Trail begins at the Continental Divide and immediately accesses the high alpine region of the park, providing up-close views of 9,000-foot peaks and snowfields that melt into meadows of wildflowers. This is one of the most loved trails in Montana and is seldom free of summer visitors, for good reason. Mountain goats seem to pose for the camera, and wildflowers change the scenery from brilliant yellow glacier lilies in June to purple aster, sticky geranium, Indian paintbrush, and mountain gentian before the fall foliage flash of August's first frost.

Best Time

The trail opening coincides with the Going-to-the-Sun Road snow clearing over Logan Pass, usually in mid-June, and it remains open into October; the parking lot is often full 11 a.m.–3 p.m., but the shuttle runs regularly.

Finding the Trail

From the summit of Going-to-the-Sun Road at Logan Pass, the trailhead is behind/west of the Logan Pass Visitor Center. A wheelchair-accessible ramp between the parking lot and trailhead encourages access to the visitor center and the initial 0.35-mile paved trail section. Snow may limit how far the trail is safely passable. The trail is occasionally closed for bear activity. Pay attention to signage.

TRAIL USE
Day hiking, child-friendly

LENGTH
5.14 miles, 2–4 hours

VERTICAL FEET
±485' to overlook and another ±787' to lake

DIFFICULTY
1 **2** 3 4 5

TRAIL TYPE
Out-and-back

SURFACE TYPE
Pavement, boardwalk, dirt, and snow

START & END
N48° 41.727'
W113° 43.102'

FEATURES
Lake
Flora
Geologic Interest
Historic Interest
Wildlife

FACILITIES
Restrooms
Bookstore
Interpretive center
Shuttle

Trail Description

Wildlife

The above-treeline trek begins at 6,646 feet elevation and climbs quickly over 1.4 miles to the Hidden Lake Overlook—a challenge for those not used to the elevation. Look for ermine, mountain goats, bighorn sheep, and skiers. Before the snow melts from the skirt of Clements Mountain, skiers and snowboarders will climb the snowfield for summer schussing. Depending on the amount of snow, the trail may be slippery or mushy. A hiking pole is handy. The intense winter weather damages the trail so that some portions are rebuilt, resulting in trail detours or closures. A boardwalk makes for easy hiking and is in place to protect the fragile plants until you reach the glacial moraine near the trail's summit.

Hidden Lake was called Bearhat Lake, or *Nupqu-kayuka,* by Kootenai Indians and drains via dramatic waterfalls into Avalanche Creek.

From the overlook, visitors see dramatic examples of glaciation, which occurred during the last ice age ending some 10,000 years ago. The geology here reveals layers of sedimentary rock, remnants of the ancient Belt Sea. You'll see evidence in ripple marks in the red argillite rock underfoot.

Geologic Interest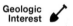

Hidden Lake seems to wrap around 8,684-foot Bearhat Mountain and is indeed crescent-shaped. The prominent peak just south is 9,125-foot Reynolds Mountain, neighbor to 8,760-foot Clements Mountain and 8,180-foot Mount Oberlin.

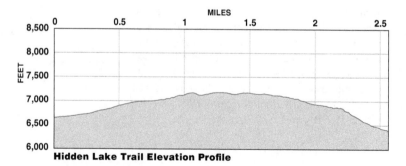

Hidden Lake Trail Elevation Profile

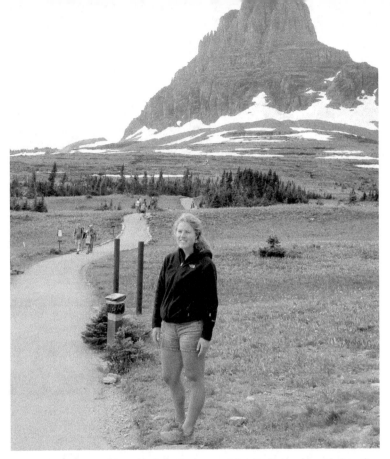

The initial 0.35 mile *of the Hidden Lake Trail is paved, but the climb to the overlook can be challenging for those not used to the elevation.*

Most people turn around at the overlook, but there's another 1.17 miles of trail down to the lake itself. If you decide to go beyond the overlook, note that several game trails weave westward. The trail crews placed logs and brush over these trails to encourage people to stay on the main route down to the lake. It's steep enough that four switchbacks zig and zag to descend 600 feet in the final half mile to the lake's 6,385 feet elevation.

The park service requests that hikers stay on the boardwalk and trail to avoid damaging the delicate floral banquet. Be on the lookout for small mammals, including ermine, Columbian ground squirrels, and chipmunks.

Lake   The reward is a frigid turquoise lake full of trout and occasional icebergs—President George H. W. Bush hiked and fished here in 1983, when he was vice president. Several large flat stepping-stone rocks are just under the surface along the northwest corner of the lake, perfect for cooling the toes.

🚶 MILESTONES

▶1   0.0   Start from the Logan Pass Visitor Center.
▶2   0.35 Pavement ends.
▶3   1.4   Hidden Lake Overlook
▶4   2.57 Hidden Lake. Return to visitor center.

Highline Trail to Granite Park Chalet (along the Garden Wall)

Hikers will encounter plenty of wildlife on the Highline Trail, one of the most loved trails in Glacier. Look for inquisitive mountain goats and whistling hoary marmots. Golden eagles soar high above, riding late summer thermals. Grizzly bears traipse here, too; be prepared by hiking in groups, making noise, and packing bear spray—and knowing how to use the bear deterrent.

Best Time

The trail opens after snow melts from the Logan Pass portion of the route, usually late June, and once the National Park Service trail crew deems the trail passable. On hot summer days, it is best traveled in early morning—few trees shade the trail.

Finding the Trail

From the Logan Pass Visitor Center, walk north across Going-to-the-Sun Road at the well-marked crosswalk. Use extreme caution when crossing the road. Follow the path 0.25 mile through the small meadow to the trailhead sign. Parking is limited at Logan Pass; a free shuttle service provides transportation from several locations, including the Apgar Transit Center, where plenty of parking is available.

Trail Description

The Highline Trail immediately accesses the high-alpine landscape yet with little elevation gain from the 6,646-foot elevation of Logan Pass. Panoramic

TRAIL USE
Day hiking,
youth-friendly

LENGTH
15.2 miles, 6–8 hours

VERTICAL FEET
±207'

DIFFICULTY
1 **2 3** 4 5

TRAIL TYPE
Out-and-back

SURFACE TYPE
Dirt and gravel

START & END
N48° 41.796'
W113° 43.088'

FEATURES
Flora
Secluded
Geologic Interest
Historic Interest
Wildlife
Views

FACILITIES
Ranger station
Interpretive center
Campgrounds
Backcountry chalet
Shuttle

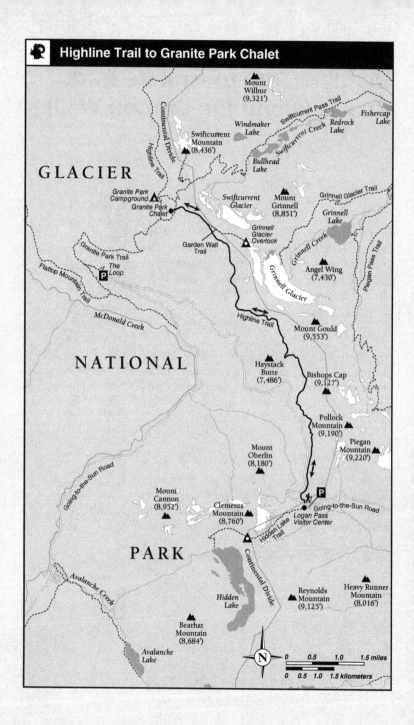

Mount
Wilbur
(9,321')

Windmaker
Lake

Swiftcurrent Pass Trail

Swiftcurrent Creek

Redrock
Lake

Fishercap
Lake

Continental Divide

Highline Trail

Swiftcurrent
Mountain
(8,436')

Bullhead
Lake

GLACIER

Granite Park
Campground

Swiftcurrent
Glacier

Mount
Grinnell
(8,851')

Grinnell Glacier Trail

Grinnell
Lake

Granite Park
Chalet

Grinnell
Glacier
Overlook

Garden Wall
Trail

Grinnell Creek

Angel Wing
(7,430')

Granite Park Trail

The Loop

Flattop Mountain Trail

P

Grinnell Glacier

Piegan Pass Trail

McDonald Creek

NATIONAL

Highline Trail

Mount Gould
(9,553')

Haystack
Butte
(7,486')

Bishops Cap
(9,127')

Pollock
Mountain
(9,190')

Piegan
Mountain
(9,220')

Mount
Oberlin
(8,180')

Going-to-the-Sun Road

Mount
Cannon
(8,952')

Clements
Mountain
(8,760')

P

Logan Pass
Visitor Center

Going-to-the-Sun Road

Hidden Lake Trail

PARK

Continental Divide

Avalanche Creek

Hidden
Lake

Reynolds
Mountain
(9,125')

Heavy Runner
Mountain
(8,016')

Bearhat
Mountain
(8,684')

Avalanche
Lake

N

0   0.5   1.0   1.5 miles

0   0.5   1.0   1.5 kilometers

OPTIONS

If you don't feel like retracing your steps to Logan Pass, you can connect to the Loop Trail for the optional hike to the Loop on Going-to-the-Sun Road (see Trail 18 for full details; shuttle required).

views of the Livingston and Lewis mountain ranges provide continual backdrops throughout the route.

After crossing the flower-strewn Logan Pass meadow, the trail hugs the rimrock of Piegan Mountain. The trail here was blasted out of the rock. A "handrail" cable, bolted to the rock wall, offers some confidence for hikers because this 0.2 mile allows cliffside exposure. The trail parallels the Continental Divide above and Going-to-the-Sun Road below.

 Views

The trail descends slightly across boulder fields and meadow areas. As soon as the snow melts, brilliant yellow glacier lilies sprout and bloom, carpeting the meadows. Above, bighorn sheep browse for shrubs and grasses, seeking minerals from naturally occurring salt licks. You might hear marmots before you see them scurrying among the rocks. Look back toward the trailhead, and you see Mount Cannon, Mount Oberlin, and Clements Mountains.

 Flora

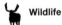 Wildlife

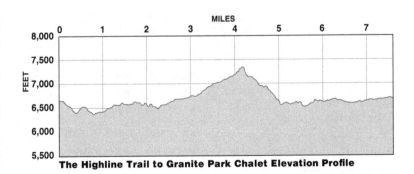

The Highline Trail to Granite Park Chalet Elevation Profile

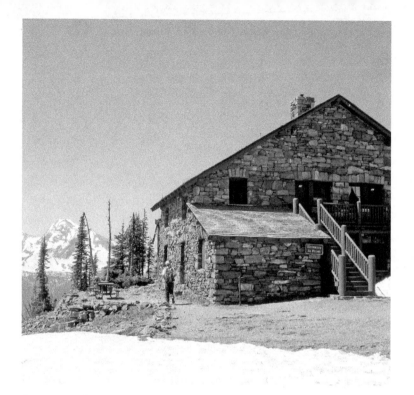

Granite Park Chalet *opened in 1914 and still offers rustic lodging.*

Secluded

For an incredible backcountry stay, book a night at the 1914 Granite Park Chalet (**granitepark chalet.com**), operated as a hikers hut with simple accommodations yet outstanding memories.

The farther you hike, the fewer humans you encounter—most people turn around in the first mile, yet the rewards of continuing are many: wildflowers; huckleberries; and lunch on large, flat "picnic rocks" in a saddle between 7,486-foot Haystack Butte and 9,553-foot Mount Gould, the highest elevation point of the Garden Wall.

For an incredible panoptic view, climb the spur route to the Grinnell Glacier Overlook (a 1.1-mile round-trip), departing from the trail at 6.8 miles and scrambling up the Garden Wall Trail to the Continental Divide. You'll want your windbreaker, water bottle, and camera—views include the Many Glacier Valley and the retreating Grinnell Glacier, as well as the plains to the east and Lake McDonald Valley to the west.

The famous Night of the Grizzlies, now a book and a documentary, occurred just below Granite Park Chalet when, in 1967, an off-duty park concession employee was dragged from her sleeping bag, mauled, and killed, despite heroic efforts of chalet and campground guests to save her. A visitor was mauled and killed the same night by a different grizzly bear at Trout Lake, some 10 air miles southwest.

Granite Park Chalet is the turnaround point to retrace your steps to Logan Pass, although the trail continues north toward Goat Haunt Ranger Station and Waterton Township, Canada, some 22 rugged miles—passports required. The chalet, open late June to early September, sells snacks. Lodging is usually fully booked months in advance. Nearby composting toilets are open to the public.

Historic Interest

🚶 MILESTONES

►1	0.0	Start from Logan Pass Visitor Center.
►2	0.01	Cross Going-to-the-Sun Road at the crosswalk.
►3	0.25	Trailhead signpost
►4	3.58	Haystack
►5	6.8	Garden Wall Trail spur to Grinnell Glacier Overlook
►6	7.6	Granite Park Chalet. Return to visitor center.

Going-to-the-Sun Road, completed in 1933, was named for a Blackfeet deity, Sour Spirit, who traveled from the sun to teach hunting. Sour Spirit's image is on Going-to-the-Sun Mountain.

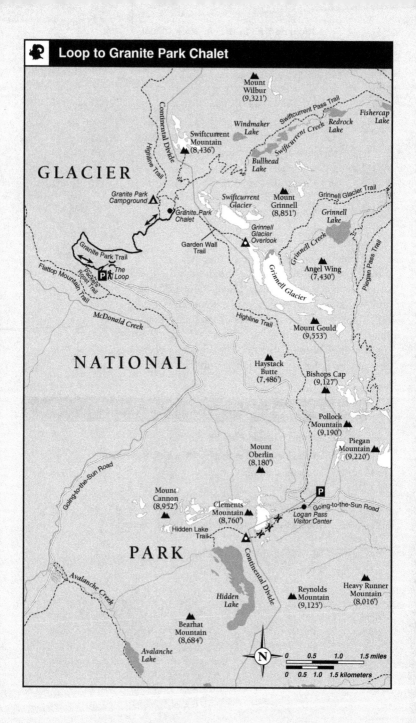

GLACIER

NATIONAL

PARK

Mount Wilbur (9,321')

Windmaker Lake

Swiftcurrent Pass Trail

Fishercap Lake

Swiftcurrent Mountain (8,436')

Swiftcurrent Creek

Redrock Lake

Continental Divide

Highline Trail

Bullhead Lake

Granite Park Campground

Swiftcurrent Glacier

Mount Grinnell (8,851')

Grinnell Glacier Trail

Granite Park Chalet

Grinnell Lake

Grinnell Glacier Overlook

Grinnell Creek

Granite Park Trail

Garden Wall Trail

Fischer's Loop Trail

The Loop

Grinnell Glacier

Angel Wing (7,430')

Piegan Pass Trail

Flattop Mountain Trail

McDonald Creek

Highline Trail

Mount Gould (9,553')

Haystack Butte (7,486')

Bishops Cap (9,127')

Pollock Mountain (9,190')

Piegan Mountain (9,220')

Mount Oberlin (8,180')

Going-to-the-Sun Road

Mount Cannon (8,952')

Clements Mountain (8,760')

Logan Pass Visitor Center

Going-to-the-Sun Road

Hidden Lake Trail

Continental Divide

Avalanche Creek

Hidden Lake

Bearhat Mountain (8,684')

Reynolds Mountain (9,125')

Heavy Runner Mountain (8,016')

Avalanche Lake

N

0   0.5   1.0   1.5 miles

0   0.5 1.0   1.5 kilometers

Loop Trail to Granite Park Chalet

Since the 2003 Trapper Creek Fire cleared much of the lodgepole pine forest, the Loop Trail now allows superb views nearly the entire way. Extensive wildflowers, such as columbine, Indian paintbrush, and fireweed, carpet the 2,200-foot elevation gain to Granite Park Chalet. The standing dead trees are bleaching white, offering a unique glimpse at fire ecology—the rebirth of a forest is in full bloom. Great horned owls, mountain bluebirds, and pileated woodpeckers perch on the dead trees.

Note: Be sure to pack water—there is no water at the trailhead. Water is available for sale at the chalet, which is open late June to early September. Because much of the trail is exposed to intense sun or weather, be sure to dress and pack for a variety of temperatures.

Best Time

It's best to go in June and July. While snow keeps the Highline Trail closed, the Loop Trail provides access to Granite Park Chalet. Once the Highline Trail opens mid-July, most hikers begin at Logan Pass, hike the gentler but longer Highline to Granite Park Chalet, and descend along the Loop Trail.

Finding the Trail

From Going-to-the-Sun Road, the Loop Trail begins on the west side of Logan Pass at the Loop parking area. Use caution when crossing the road to the trailhead just west of the road's sharp turn,

TRAIL USE
Day hiking,
youth-friendly

LENGTH
8.4 miles, 4–6 hours

VERTICAL FEET
±2,200'

DIFFICULTY
1 2 3 **4** 5

TRAIL TYPE
Out-and-back

SURFACE TYPE
Dirt

START & END
N48° 45.299'
W113° 48.030'

FEATURES
Flora
Secluded
Geologic Interest
Historic Interest
Views
Photo opportunity
Wildfire ecology

FACILITIES
Shuttle
Campsites
Chalet
Limited food and water
for sale
Clovis composting
toilets

133

Geologic Interest

Historic Interest

"The Loop." Large signs reveal the trailhead, which departs behind roadside boulders and a rock wall.

Trail Description

The trail leads north for 0.1 mile, then crosses a roaring creek via a wooden footbridge. After crossing the footbridge, look south to the massive Heaven's Peak, 8,967 feet tall. The park's geology is etched in Heaven's Peak's layers of rock. When snow covers the peak, you can see why the American Indians call this the Land of the Shining Mountains. You may encounter horse-pack trains hauling supplies to Granite Park Chalet—give the equines the trail, and talk gently so they may pass without trouble.

As the trail switchbacks, the new view is east toward Logan Pass and provides glimpses of 8,952-foot Mount Cannon and 8,180-foot Mount Oberlin, with its 500-foot-long Bird Woman Falls draping the northern shoulder. The falls are probably named for the Blackfeet Indian Bird Woman, the wife of Lone Walker. You will see flashes of Going-to-the-Sun Road and solid views of the Garden Wall, a glacial arête marking the Continental Divide. Below is a fine example of glaciated valley, the U shape carved by thousands of years of glaciers moving over the rock to form McDonald Creek and McDonald Lake.

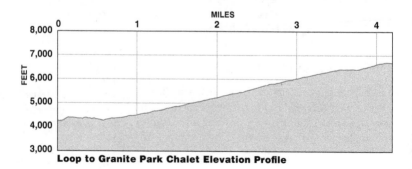

Loop to Granite Park Chalet Elevation Profile

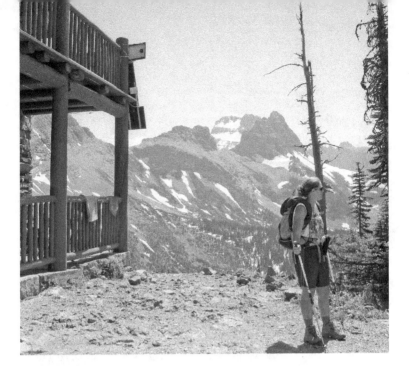

Granite Park Chalet's *decks overlook the Garden Wall to the south.*

At the 3-mile mark, the forest greens up because the 2003 fires skipped over this area. There is more shade, and often patches of snow even into late July, as the trail levels out and approaches the campground. Beargrass and huckleberry bushes line the trail at the junction of the Granite Park Campground, scene of the notorious 1967 Night of the Grizzlies incident, in which a Glacier Park concession employee was dragged out of her sleeping bag and killed by a grizzly bear. Another woman met a similar fate miles away at Trout Lake. Both occurred

 Flora

 Camping

If weather permits, hikers can connect to the Highline Trail (see Trail 17 for details) for a one-way hike.

the same August night and were made famous in Jack Olsen's book *Night of the Grizzlies.* This sobering note is a reminder to hike in groups, make plenty of noise, and carry a canister of bear spray.

Views

You will cross a shallow creek just before the final climb to Granite Park Chalet—the "granite" is a misnomer: The rock is a basalt called Purcell lava. Lunch on the deck offers nearly 360 degrees of incredible views. Note that some cell phones receive service in the chalet area.

MILESTONES

▶1 0.0 Start from the Loop parking area.

▶2 0.1 Bridge crossing

▶3 0.6 Packers' Roost junction; follow the Loop Trail to the right/northeast to the chalet.

▶4 3.66 Granite Park Campground junction and pit toilet

▶5 4.2 Granite Park Chalet. Return to parking area.

Siyeh Bend Trail and Piegan Pass Trail (Siyeh Bend to Jackson Glacier Overlook)

The Siyeh Bend Trail connects to the Piegan Pass Trail for an easy half-loop route that is below the snow line by late spring, when Going-to-the Sun Road may not be completely open to Logan Pass. This trip is perfect for hikers who don't wish to wait for Logan Pass to open before getting into the backcountry.

Best Time

The trail is mostly snow-free by mid- to late June and offers considerable shade for hot summer days. Access to Going-to-the-Sun Road dictates availability dates for trailhead access, generally through early October.

Finding the Trail

From Going-to-the-Sun Road at Siyeh Bend (2.2 miles east of Logan Pass), look for the large sign for Piegan Pass immediately behind the road's rock wall. This is also the trailhead to access the Siyeh Pass Trail and Piegan Pass Trail. It's easiest to park at Jackson Glacier Overlook and ride the westbound shuttle to the shuttle stop at Siyeh Bend.

Trail Description

The Siyeh Bend Trail initially leads north and upstream alongside Siyeh Creek for 0.1 mile before snaking upward and south. The spectacular scenery punctuated with beargrass and huckleberry at trail's beginning gives way to a brief climb into thick

TRAIL USE
Day hiking, child-friendly

LENGTH
2.5 miles, 2–3 hours

VERTICAL FEET
±870'

DIFFICULTY
1 **2** 3 4 5

TRAIL TYPE
Point-to-point

SURFACE TYPE
Dirt and gravel

START
N48° 42.092'
W113° 40.046'

END
N48° 40.660'
W113° 39.156'

FEATURES
Flora
Secluded
Geologic Interest
Historic Interest
Wildlife
Birds
Views

FACILITIES
Phone
Ranger station
Lodging, Restaurants
Stores, Gas
Interpretive center
Shuttle

137

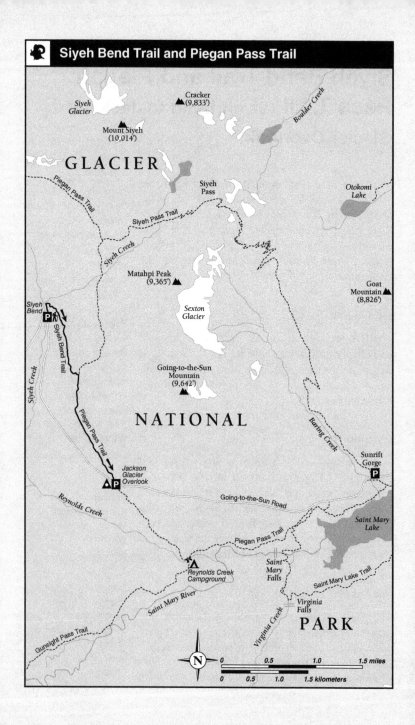

GLACIER

Siyeh
Glacier

Cracker
(9,833')

Boulder Creek

Mount Siyeh
(10,014')

Siyeh
Pass

Otokomi
Lake

Piegan Pass Trail

Siyeh Pass Trail

Siyeh Creek

Matahpi Peak
(9,365')

Goat
Mountain
(8,826')

Sexton
Glacier

Siyeh
Bend

P

Siyeh Bend Trail

Going-to-the-Sun
Mountain
(9,642')

NATIONAL

Siyeh Creek

Piegan Pass Trail

Baring Creek

Sunrift
Gorge
P

Jackson Glacier
Overlook

P

Going-to-the-Sun Road

Reynolds Creek

Saint Mary
Lake

Piegan Pass Trail

Reynolds Creek
Campground

Saint
Mary
Falls

Saint Mary Lake Trail

Saint Mary River

Virginia Creek

Virginia
Falls

PARK

Gunsight Pass Trail

N

0   0.5   1.0   1.5 miles

0   0.5   1.0   1.5 kilometers

spruce and pine trees yet soon provides an easy and mostly downhill route not far above Going-to-the-Sun Road, one that affords a few patches of snow in the shade through June. Until recently, the route offered limited views, but after a huge avalanche in winter 2011 swept down the shoulders of Piegan Mountain, across the valley, and up the other side, trees that obstructed views are now splintered, snapped, or demolished. During the avalanche, trees were severed 6 to 12 feet from the ground, leaving debris covering the meadows and trail. The trail crew has cleared the trail—a never-ending job, as each year trees fall across the park's nearly 750 miles of trail with or without the help of avalanches.

Look east for glimpses of Going-to-the-Sun Mountain. Look to the south across the valley for a glimpse at Blackfoot Glacier. Glacier National Park's archives include a 1914 photograph showing Blackfoot and Jackson Glaciers cojoined. Today, the shrinking glaciers have retreated to their own cirques. From this vantage, it's easy to see how the glaciers carved valleys. Snow and ice accumulated over centuries, and the weight of the accumulation caused the compacted ice—a glacier—to move, scraping the rock and soil underneath. After thousands of years of glacial advance and retreat, the landscape is one of serrated mountains and deep, U-shaped valleys.

Siyeh comes from the Blackfeet word *saiyi,* meaning wild, mad, or rabid, as in a mad wolf.

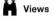 Views

Geologic Interest

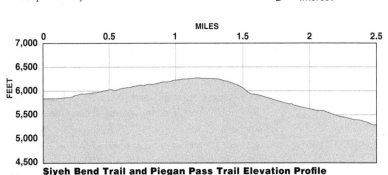

Siyeh Bend Trail and Piegan Pass Trail Elevation Profile

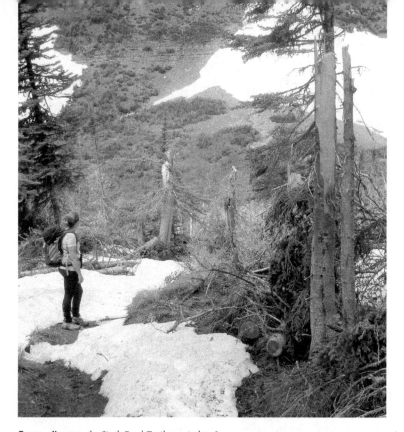

Snow clings *to the Siyeh Bend Trail even in late June.*

Soon, the trail enters a spruce and fir forest, which at times is quite dense. Here, you may hear birds, such as the pine grosbeak, with its rosy head, back, and rump, and the red crossbill, more orange than red and named because its mandibles are crossed at the tips to enable easy seed extraction from pinecones. Delicate, shade-loving flowers thrive here, too, such as shooting star and meadow rue, a plant easily confused with columbine as the leaves are similar but with distinctly different flowers. Some American Indians used fragrant meadow rue as a perfume.

The Siyeh Formation, a dolomite and limestone rock, is visible in this part of the park. Some portions display fossil algae in rosette shapes; these are

Birds

Flora

The Piegan Pass Trail is part of the Continental Divide National Scenic Trail, which wends about 3,100 miles across five states and three national parks. Some 980 miles pass through Montana, of which 110 are within Glacier National Park.

from the Proterozoic Eon, the later Precambrian time, some 2.5 billion to 570 million years ago. The rosette-shaped fossil algae can be seen along Going-to-the-Sun Road near Logan Pass at mile 23.7 (from West Glacier).

After meeting the junction with the Piegan Pass Trail and heading right/south and down, you will encounter four switchbacks dropping 870 feet in elevation en route to Going-to-the-Sun Road and Jackson Glacier Overlook. Hiking poles are handy for people whose knees don't appreciate a speedy descent.

MILESTONES

▶1	0.0	Start from Siyeh Bend on Going-to-the-Sun Road, 2.2 miles east of Logan Pass.
▶2	0.1	Trail leaves the creek side and turns left/east and uphill for a brief climb.
▶3	1.2	Junction with Piegan Pass Trail; take the right/south fork down to Jackson Glacier Overlook.
▶4	2.5	Jackson Glacier Overlook on Going-to-the-Sun Road

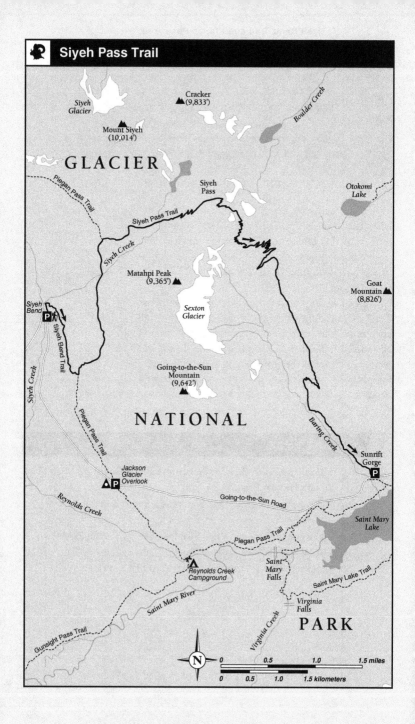

Siyeh Glacier

Cracker
(9,833')

Mount Siyeh
(10,014')

Boulder Creek

GLACIER

Piegan Pass Trail

Siyeh Pass

Otokomi Lake

Siyeh Pass Trail

Siyeh Creek

Matahpi Peak
(9,365')

Sexton Glacier

Goat Mountain
(8,826')

Siyeh Bend

Siyeh Bend Trail

Going-to-the-Sun Mountain
(9,642')

NATIONAL

Piegan Pass Trail

Baring Creek

Sunrift Gorge

Jackson Glacier Overlook

Going-to-the-Sun Road

Reynolds Creek

Saint Mary Lake

Piegan Pass Trail

Saint Mary Lake Trail

Reynolds Creek Campground

Saint Mary Falls

Saint Mary River

Virginia Falls

PARK

Gunsight Pass Trail

Virginia Creek

N

| 0 | 0.5 | 1.0 | 1.5 miles |
| 0 | 0.5 | 1.0 | 1.5 kilometers |

Siyeh Pass Trail
(Siyeh Bend to Sunrift Gorge)

Siyeh Pass is one of the most spectacular hikes in Glacier and is among local hikers' favorites. The route begins in a flower-filled valley, crosses through spruce and subalpine fir forest, climbs to a meadow, and travels within sight of the terminal moraine at Sexton Glacier. Mountain goats, bighorn sheep, and grizzly and black bears live here—carry bear spray. Snow hazards exist on the trail's upper realms. The trail is more difficult until the snow melts from the pass area. Check with the ranger station to see if crampons and ice axes are needed for midsummer snow crossing or if a hiking pole is sufficient. The hike finishes at the narrow slot canyon of Sunrift Gorge, where centuries of crushing waters have scoured smooth the red argillite on the gorge's walls.

Best Time

The trail becomes snow-free in late July and remains a fantastic route through mid-October or until the first snow falls. Check with rangers regarding the icy snow crossing at the pass. Watch for trail closures due to bear activity.

Finding the Trail

From Going-to-the-Sun Road at Siyeh Bend (2.2 miles east of Logan Pass), look for the large sign for Piegan Pass immediately behind the road's rock wall. This is also the trailhead to access the Siyeh Pass Trail and Piegan Pass Trail. It's easiest to park at Sunrift Gorge (7 miles east of Logan Pass) and

TRAIL USE
Day hiking

LENGTH
10.3 miles, 6–8 hours

VERTICAL FEET
+3,395'/-4,561'

DIFFICULTY
1 2 3 **4 5**

TRAIL TYPE
Point-to-point

SURFACE TYPE
Dirt, gravel, rock, snow, and ice

START
N48° 42.092'
W113° 40.046'

END
N48° 40.709'
W113° 35.721'

FEATURES
Flora
Geologic Interest
Historic Interest
Wildlife
Birds
Views

FACILITIES
Ranger station
Lodging, Restaurants
Stores, Gas
Interpretive center
Campgrounds
Shuttle

ride the westbound shuttle up to the shuttle stop at
Siyeh Bend.

Trail Description

The Siyeh Bend Trail initially leads north and
upstream alongside Siyeh Creek for 0.1 mile before
snaking up and south. At 1.2 miles, just after a
creek crossing, the trail meets Piegan Pass Trail;
take the left/north course. Soon the trail climbs
above the trees and into a beautiful meadow, Preston Park. Look for the junction to the right/east
with Siyeh Pass Trail. From here, it's a climb to the
pass. The rewards are many: glacial tarns, waterfalls, and views of Piegan Glacier and Piegan Pass.
You also get a spectacular view of Mount Siyeh
ahead; over your shoulder, you see Cataract, Pollock, Reynolds, and Piegan Mountains.

The saddle provides yet more views—but hold
on to your gear; powerful winds buffet the mountain and can steal your belongings. Those afternoon thermals also carry migrants on wing. Each
fall, hundreds of golden eagles ride the thermals
from northern Canada's breeding grounds to Mexico's winter respite—and retrace the flight each
spring. Notably, female golden eagles are larger
than the males, with a 7-foot wingspan, and often

Flora

Views

Birds

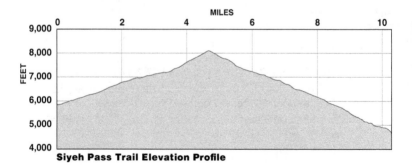

Siyeh Pass Trail Elevation Profile

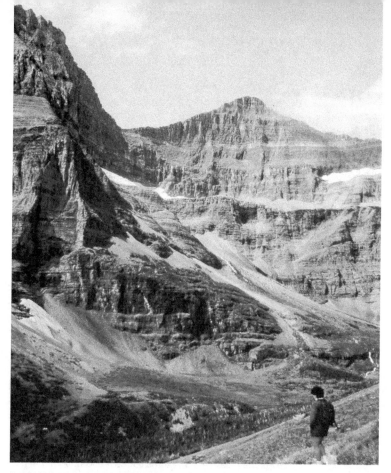

At 7,911 feet, *Siyeh Pass is the highest trail elevation pass in Glacier and often remains encased in snow until mid-July.*

circle for a time waiting for their smaller mates to catch up. Don't forget to look at the deep crevasses in Sexton Glacier below Matahpi Peak and Going-to-the-Sun Mountain. An unmarked trail accesses Sexton Glacier.

Over the next 5.5 miles, the trail descends 3,450 feet, initially down a series of switchbacks, where mountain goats might challenge your passage—give them wide berth. Despite their curious appearance, they are wild and unpredictable ungulates, known to charge hikers who get too close.

 Wildlife

NOTES

Look up to Mount Siyeh. At 10,014 feet, the peak—the park's fifth tallest—is often summited, but the north face of Siyeh was successfully climbed only once, in 1979, after two men spent three days on the rock wall and two nights bivouacked on the rock.

Geologic Interest ✦

Little Chief Mountain frames the view as the trail cruises the alpine region until it descends into a forested gorge, noisy from cascading streams foaming off the red rock walls. In the final mile, you'll encounter more hikers, up from Going-to-the-Sun Road through Sunrift Gorge. Baring Creek's speedy plunge has smoothed the rock walls to resemble an amusement park waterslide—don't be tempted to swim here as the dangers are many, from frigid water temperatures to crushing rock walls and waterfalls.

🚶 MILESTONES

▶1   0.0   Start from Siyeh Bend on Going-to-the-Sun Road, 2.2 miles east of Logan Pass on the Siyeh Bend Trail, aka Piegan Pass Trail and Siyeh Pass route.

▶2   0.1   Trail leaves the creek side and turns left/east and up for a brief climb.

▶3   1.2   Junction with Piegan Pass Trail; take left/north fork toward Piegan Pass and Siyeh Pass.

▶4   2.6   Junction with Siyeh Pass Trail

▶5   4.7   Siyeh Pass

▶6   10.3   Sunrift Gorge at Going-to-the-Sun Road

CAUTION

Don't pick the flowers! Preston Park is an especially verdant subalpine meadow of showy blossoms, wildflowers that must retain their root systems and seeds for future seasons. Picking or taking any part of a plant is prohibited by the park service.

Piegan Pass Trail

Piegan Pass Trail is a perfect introduction to the high-country passes for fit hikers who are acclimatized to elevation and the rarefied air near the Continental Divide. The trail begins at 6,315 feet elevation and provides a continuous yet gentle climb to Piegan Pass at 7,565 feet elevation. The route wraps through subalpine fir and spruce forest before climbing near the treeline and into flower-filled meadows. A snow crossing challenges visitors well into August—a hiking pole is handy. Grand views of Piegan Mountain and Piegan Glacier line the ascent to the west and Matahpi Peak, Mount Siyeh, and Cataract Mountain to the east and north. The climb finishes in a saddle pass with more grand views of the Many Glacier Valley.

Best Time

Snow melts from the trail by mid-July, although a few patches of snow remain well into August. The trailhead is accessible from the time Going-to-the-Sun Road opens to Siyeh Bend by mid-June until snow closes the road in October. Watch for trail closures due to bear activity.

Finding the Trail

From Going-to-the-Sun Road at Siyeh Bend (2.2 miles east of Logan Pass), look for the large sign for Piegan Pass immediately behind the road's rock wall. This is also the trailhead to access the Siyeh Pass Trail. Since parking is limited, hikers are

TRAIL USE
Day hiking

LENGTH
9.0 miles, 4–6 hours

VERTICAL FEET
±1,742'

DIFFICULTY
1 2 **3** 4 5

TRAIL TYPE
Out-and-back

SURFACE TYPE
Dirt, gravel, rock, snow, and ice

START & END
N48° 42.092'
W113° 40.046'

FEATURES
Flora
Secluded
Geologic Interest
Historic Interest
Wildlife
Glacier

FACILITIES
Ranger station
Lodging
Restaurants
Stores
Gas
Interpretive center
Campgrounds
Shuttle

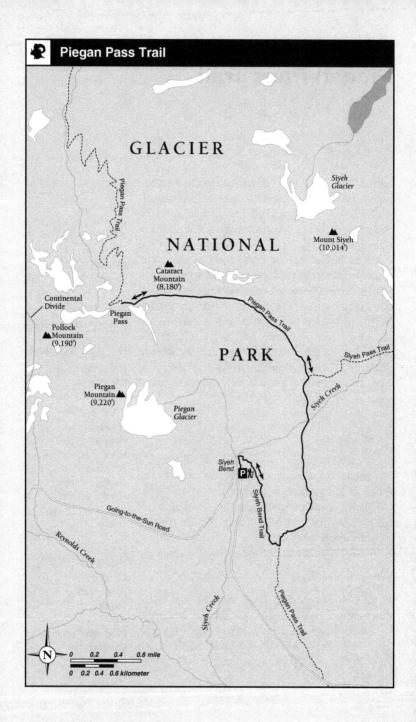

Piegan Pass Trail

GLACIER

NATIONAL

PARK

Siyeh Glacier

▲ Mount Siyeh
(10,014')

Piegan Pass Trail

▲ Cataract Mountain
(8,180')

Continental Divide

Piegan Pass

▲ Pollock Mountain
(9,190')

Siyeh Pass Trail

Siyeh Creek

▲ Piegan Mountain
(9,220')

Piegan Glacier

Siyeh Bend

P

Siyeh Bend Trail

Going-to-the-Sun Road

Piegan Pass Trail

Reynolds Creek

Siyeh Creek

N

0   0.2   0.4   0.6 mile
0 0.2 0.4 0.6 kilometer

encouraged to ride the free shuttle to Siyeh Bend—check locally for the daily shuttle schedule.

Trail Description

The trailhead at Siyeh Bend provides a panorama of much of the hike ahead, directly north above the valley. Along the right, the skirt of 10,014-foot Mount Siyeh, the trail crosses scree, snow, and minimal vegetation. Initially, however, the route follows the Siyeh Bend Trail in the opposite direction and through the path of a 2011 avalanche. The snow mass crashed down the west flank of Piegan Mountain and splashed up the east side of the valley, snapping 18-inch-thick trees in two.

The trail climbs slightly as it runs south through the forest, rife with deer, elk, chipmunks, and ground squirrels. Look for shade-loving flowers, such as the rare mountain lady's slipper. After crossing small footbridges, the junction with Piegan Pass Trail at 1.2 miles intersects; a left/northeast turn leads toward Piegan Pass. A right/southwest trek heads down 1.3 miles to Going-to-the-Sun Road at Jackson Glacier Overlook—an alternative trailhead for the Piegan Pass hike with an additional 1,400 vertical feet.

> The glaciers viewed from this trail include the 60-acre Piegan Glacier, 440-acre Blackfoot Glacier, and 250-acre Jackson Glacier.

 Wildlife

 Flora

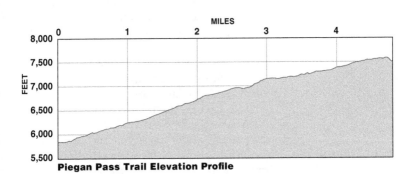

Piegan Pass Trail Elevation Profile

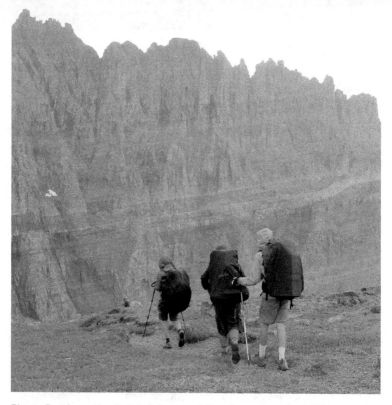

Piegan Pass's gentle climb *includes views of three glaciers, astonishing wildflowers, and often patches of August snow.*

An impressive log bridge provides views of Piegan Mountain. From here, the forest opens up into meadows of Indian paintbrush, beargrass, asters, and the showy death camas, which lives up to its name. From the junction with Siyeh Pass at 2.6 miles, the subalpine trees and aspens thin, finally giving way to the scree-lined trail as seen from the parking area below. The final mile provides some exposure; however, it's the snow crossing that may deter hikers if conditions are icy.

Wildflowers

Once above the treeline, Piegan Glacier becomes visible immediately west. Look south to see the park's largest glacier, Blackfoot, and its neighbor, Jackson Glacier. Ahead, the saw-toothed arête of the Garden Wall looms above Piegan Pass.

Glacier

NOTES

Piegan Pass, Mountain, and Glacier are named for the Piegan Indians, one of three main branches of the Blackfeet Confederacy and whose 3,000-square-mile Blackfeet Nation is due east of Glacier National Park.

Like many of Glacier's trails, Piegan Pass Trail has alternatives to lengthen the hike and increase the viewshed, including hiking beyond the pass and down to Many Glacier Lodge, 12.85 total miles point to point.

MILESTONES

►1	0.0	Start from Siyeh Bend on Going-to-the-Sun Road, 2.2 miles east of Logan Pass on the Siyeh Bend Trail, aka Piegan Pass Trail and Siyeh Pass route.
►2	0.1	Trail leaves the creek side and turns left/east and up for a brief climb.
►3	1.2	Junction with Piegan Pass Trail; take left/north fork toward Piegan Pass and Siyeh Pass.
►4	2.6	Junction with Siyeh Pass Trail
►5	4.5	Piegan Pass. Return to trailhead.

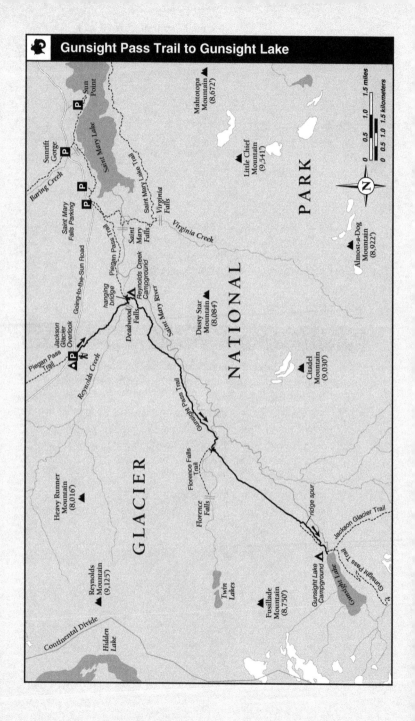

Gunsight Pass Trail to Gunsight Lake

Gunsight Pass Trail to Gunsight Lake

As one of the premier hikes in the park, the route to Gunsight Lake passes through shaded forest, along streams and waterfalls, and provides views of glaciers while traveling over hanging bridges, along cliffs, and across wildflower meadows. The trail begins at 5,182 feet elevation, drops to 4,640 in the first 1.3 miles, and then gradually climbs to 5,280 at Gunsight Lake.

Best Time

The trailhead is accessible in mid-June; however, the upper portions of the trail are hidden under snow and, in some years, deep avalanche debris until mid- or late July, making route finding difficult and the trail dangerous along cliffs. The hanging bridge at Gunsight Lake is removed/replaced seasonally—check the trail status report at **nps .gov/glac/planyourvisit/trailstatusreports.htm.** The road closes mid-October through early May.

Finding the Trail

From Going-to-the-Sun Road at 12.6 miles west of the Saint Mary Entrance Station, look for a large GUNSIGHT PASS TRAIL interpretive sign posted on the south side of the road at a large parking pull-off for Jackson Glacier Overlook. (Note that there is no vault toilet here, but there is a set of vault toilets 0.5 mile east on Going-to-the-Sun Road.) The trailhead is near the easternmost end of the parking area and on the west side of the road. The trailhead sign shows that the trail begins on the Piegan Pass Trail/ Gunsight Pass Cutoff Trail, heading downhill.

TRAIL USE
Day hiking, backpacking

LENGTH
12.6 miles, 6–9 hours

VERTICAL FEET
±1,500'

DIFFICULTY
1 2 **3** 4 5

TRAIL TYPE
Out-and-back

SURFACE TYPE
Dirt, gravel, boardwalk, snow, and ice

START & END
N48° 40.653'
W113° 39.136'

FEATURES
Flora
Geologic Interest
Historic Interest
Wildlife
Waterfalls
Lake
Fishing
Glaciers

FACILITIES
Ranger station
Lodging, Restaurants
Stores, Gas
Interpretive center
Campgrounds
Shuttle

Trail Description

Flora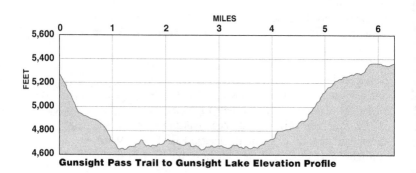

Initially, the downhill coast among thimbleberries, snowberries, and huckleberries, shaded by aspen and lodgepole pines, heads generally southeast on Gunsight Pass Cutoff Trail/Piegan Pass Trail/Continental Divide Trail. At 1.1 miles, the gushing Deadwood Falls entices photographers down a 30-foot spur to the edge of the cataract. Soon, the junction at 1.2 miles with Gunsight Pass Trail leads right/west and onto the hanging bridge over Reynolds Creek, where Reynolds Creek Campground, with three tent sites, is snug in the woods.

Waterfall

Camping

The next 2 miles cruise through patches of meadow and forest, providing glimpses of the Saint Mary River milieu, Mirror Pond, 8,084-foot Dusty Star Mountain, and 9,030-foot Citadel Mountain. A marshy environment draws common mergansers and Canada geese—the mud reveals tracks of moose, deer, bears, and beavers. At almost 4 miles, the junction with the Florence Falls Trail, a 0.6-mile spur, leads right/north to a lovely draping falls of icy water.

Wildlife

Waterfall

The final 2.3 miles to Gunsight Lake includes a 500-foot climb along an exposed cliff area lined with goldenrod and asters, and then a walk among

Gunsight Pass Trail to Gunsight Lake Elevation Profile

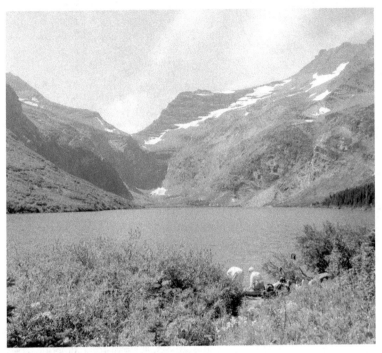

Gunsight Lake, *with Gunsight Pass in the background, is a popular destination for day hikers and backpackers.*

dead trees at the base of a massive avalanche path from 2011. Hikers first encounter the debris where a new footbridge graces a stream. It's a 0.6-mile walk through the avalanche debris, thankfully cleared by trail crews. Here, the notch between 9,258-foot Gunsight Mountain to the north and 10,052-foot Mount Jackson to the south becomes visible, and soon the lake shimmers below.

The Gunsight Lake Campground, trimmed with Engelmann spruce and subalpine firs, is one of the largest in the park, with seven tent sites, a food-prep area, food-hanging poles, two pit toilets, and stock rail. The campsites are away from the lakeshore

There are 290 named mountain passes in Montana.

▲ Camping

OPTIONS

Several options depart from Gunsight Lake, including a steep spur route up to viewpoints for Jackson and Blackfoot Glaciers with views of Citadel, Almost-a-Dog, and Logan Mountains. The continuation of the Gunsight Pass Trail climbs steeply to the 6,949-foot pass and zigzags down to Lake Ellen Wilson or on to Sperry Chalet, finishing 20.6 miles later at Lake McDonald Lodge. Note that just below Gunsight Pass are a few fairly steep snow crossings and some significant exposure, providing some thrills and danger if conditions are icy.

Lake ≋

and tucked among Engelmann spruce. While the sites mostly lack views, campers are grateful for the windbreak. A gravel beach at the foot of the 0.8- by 0.25-mile alpine lake is a perfect picnic spot.

While this discussion covers the trail to Gunsight Lake, hikers and backpackers find the entire 20.6 miles through to Lake McDonald Lodge both fantastic and strenuous. Chances are good that mid- and late-summer visitors will encounter endurance hikers speeding along the 20.6 miles all in one day and backpackers camping at Gunsight Lake, Lake Ellen Wilson, Sperry Campground, or the luxurious 1914 Sperry Chalet (reservations required). For more on the 20.6-mile point-to-point option, see the sidebar above.

🚶 MILESTONES

►1 0.0 Start from Going-to-the-Sun Road at Jackson Glacier Overlook, on the Piegan Pass Trail/Gunsight Pass Cutoff Trail, heading downhill.

►2 1.1 Spur trail to Deadwood Falls

►3 1.2 Junction with Gunsight Pass Trail and hanging bridge a bit farther

►4 1.25 Reynolds Creek Campground and pit toilet

►5 3.92 Junction with spur trail to Florence Falls and bridge over creek

►6 5.52 Turn left onto ridge spur.

►7 5.96 Rejoin Gunsight Pass Trail.

►8 6.3 Gunsight Lake and Campground. Return to trailhead.

Sun Point Nature Trail to Reynolds Creek

The trail can be hiked in either direction, but this description begins at the Jackson Glacier Overlook on the Piegan Pass Trail and travels east, ending at the spectacular Sun Point. This lovely route offers a swinging bridge; frothy waterfall; lake, mountain, and glacier views; and shuttle buses that provide options to abbreviate the hike at three access points. Visitors not acclimatized to the elevation can clip off a few miles and still ride shuttles. This trail provides excellent early-season hiking when Going-to-the-Sun Road isn't fully open and snow cloaks higher elevations.

Best Time

The trail becomes snow-free by May in most years, but the Going-to-the-Sun Road opening to Jackson Glacier Overlook dictates the availability of the westernmost portion of the trail. The park's shuttle service begins in mid-June, providing easy access to trailheads.

Finding the Trail

Leave a vehicle at the large Sun Point parking and picnic area (the GPS coordinates for the endpoint), and take the westbound shuttle. Disembark at the third shuttle stop, Jackson Glacier Overlook (12.6 miles west of the Saint Mary Entrance Station). Look for the large interpretive sign on the south side of the road describing the Gunsight Pass Trail. The trail begins behind the sign heading southeast on the Piegan Pass Trail/Gunsight Pass Cutoff Trail.

TRAIL USE
Day hiking, child-friendly

LENGTH
4.5 miles, 2–3 hours

VERTICAL FEET
±793'

DIFFICULTY
1 **2** 3 4 5

TRAIL TYPE
Point-to-point

SURFACE TYPE
Dirt and gravel

START
N48° 40.660'
W113° 39.156'

END
N48° 40.567'
W113° 34.785'

FEATURES
Flora
Geologic Interest
Historic Interest
Wildlife, Birds
Waterfall
Lake

FACILITIES
Ranger station
Lodging, Restaurants
Stores, Gas
Interpretive center
Campgrounds
Picnic area
Shuttle

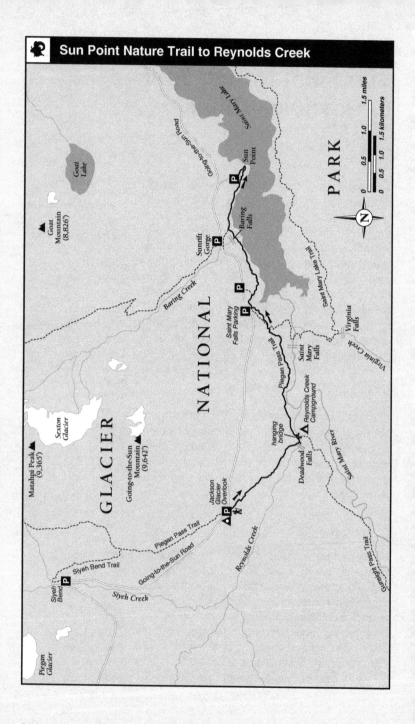

Sun Point Nature Trail to Reynolds Creek

Goat Lake

Goat Mountain (8,826')

Going-to-the-Sun Road

Saint Mary Lake

Sun Point

Baring Falls

Sunrift Gorge

Baring Creek

Saint Mary Lake Trail

Saint Mary Falls Parking

Piegan Pass Trail

Virginia Falls

Virginia Creek

Saint Mary Falls

Sexton Glacier

Reynolds Creek Campground

hanging bridge

Matahpi Peak (9,365')

Going-to-the-Sun Mountain (9,642')

Deadwood Falls

Saint Mary River

GLACIER

NATIONAL

PARK

Jackson Glacier Overlook

Piegan Pass Trail

Going-to-the-Sun Road

Reynolds Creek

Gunsight Pass Trail

Siyeh Bend Trail

Siyeh Bend

Siyeh Creek

Piegan Glacier

PARK

N

0   0.5   1.0   1.5 miles

0   0.5   1.0   1.5 kilometers

27al Tril to Reynlds Creek | TRAIL **23**

The other option is to begin at the Sun Point parking area's southeastern corner, east of the pit toilets. The trail initially heads out to Sun Point before backtracking slightly and heading west along the lakeshore.

Trail Description

Black elderberry, beargrass, and lupine favor the trailside, while sun filters through the canopy of pine, aspen, and Rocky Mountain maple. You'll pass a marshy area thick with cow parsnip—make plenty of noise here to avoid wildlife confrontations, and stay on the trail to prevent plant damage. The trail follows the Piegan Pass Trail a mile downhill, losing 660 feet in elevation and eventually meeting the frothy Reynolds Creek. Waters tumble from Logan Pass and Reynolds Mountain snows. Deadwood Falls roars in early summer—you'll hear its hydraulics before seeing the flow charging over red argillite.

 Flora

 Waterfall

Almost 0.2 mile later is the junction with Gunsight Pass Trail and the hanging bridge over Reynolds Creek—worth a trot across for photos and shaky laughs. The route to Sun Point, however, continues east on Piegan Pass Trail. As you traverse through the woods, listen for woodland birds: Mountain chickadees sing; ruffed grouse drum

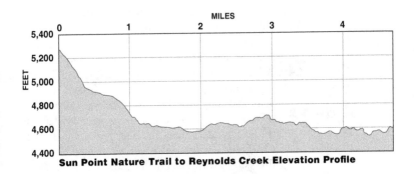

Sun Point Nature Trail to Reynolds Creek Elevation Profile

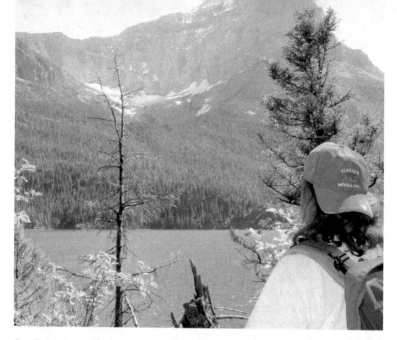

Sun Point Nature Trail *rewards hikers with incredible mountain views across Saint Mary Lake.*

Birds

Wildlife

Waterfall

Lake

wings; and magpies argue. Many mammals live here, although you might not see the bull elk, white-tailed buck, and snowshoe hare. Look for footprints in the mud that give away these shy species.

At 2.43 miles, you will encounter the junction south to Saint Mary Falls, but continue east toward Sun Point. Within a few steps will be another junction, a spur trail to the road at the Saint Mary Falls Trailhead. While this will take you to the road, it's the next spur trail that meets the Saint Mary Falls shuttle stop. Continuing to Sun Point offers rewards of scenic views en route to Baring Falls and another chance to hike up to a shuttle stop. Baring Falls is a nice picnic spot, especially if the day is breezy, since it's protected from notorious Saint Mary zephyrs. The final half mile to Sun Point provides mountain views across Saint Mary Lake as the trail wanders above the lakeshore. Citadel, Little Chief, and Going-to-the-Sun Mountains dominate the sky. Save room on the camera for Sun Point itself. The rocky promontory was once the site of the Going-to-the-Sun Chalets, summer lodging for up to 200 guests in Swiss-style cottages. Little evidence remains of the century-old chalets, other than a marker detailing the mountains in view.

 Historic Interest

🚶 MILESTONES

►1	0.0	Start from Jackson Glacier Overlook on the Piegan Pass Trail/Gunsight Pass Cutoff Trail on the south side of Going-to-the-Sun Road, hiking down and east.
►2	1.1	Deadwood Falls
►3	1.16	Junction with Gunsight Pass Trail; continue east on Piegan Pass Trail; do not cross on the hanging bridge unless you plan on camping at Reynolds Creek Campground or hiking to Gunsight Lake and Pass.
►4	2.43	Junction with Saint Mary Falls Trail; take left trail.
►5	2.45	Junction with spur route to Going-to-the-Sun Road (left/north trail); to continue to Sun Point, stay right/south.
►6	2.88	Junction with spur to Saint Mary Falls Trailhead at Going-to-the-Sun Road (left/north trail); to continue to Sun Point, stay right/south.
►7	3.5	Baring Falls and spur trail to Going-to-the-Sun Road at Sunrift Gorge (left/north trail), a 250-foot climb over 0.3 mile; to continue to Sun Point, stay right/south.
►8	4.35	Sun Point
►9	4.5	Sun Point parking area

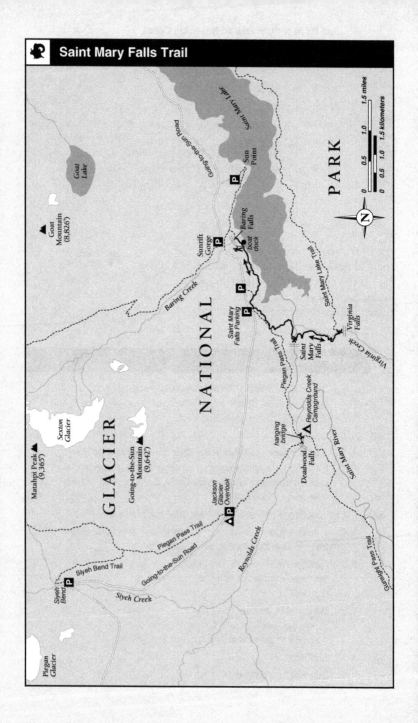

Saint Mary Falls Trail

Satin Mary Lake

Going-to-the-Sun Road

Goat Lake

Goat Mountain (8,826)

Sun Point

Baring Falls

boat dock

Sunrift Gorge

PARK

Baring Creek

Saint Mary Lake Trail

Virginia Falls

NATIONAL

Saint Mary Falls Parking

Saint Mary Falls

Virginia Creek

Plegan Pass Trail

Reynolds Creek Campground

Matahpi Peak (9,365)

Sexton Glacier

GLACIER

Going-to-the-Sun Mountain (9,642)

Jackson Glacier Overlook

hanging bridge

Deadwood Falls

Saint Mary River

Piegan Pass Trail

Going-to-the-Sun Road

Reynolds Creek

Gunsight Pass Trail

Slyeh Bend Trail

Slyeh Bend

Slyeh Creek

Piegan Glacier

Saint Mary Falls Trail

A fantastic view with every step rewards visitors to the Saint Mary Falls Trail, where a series of waterfalls sends glacial meltwater into the vibrant aquamarine Saint Mary Lake.

Best Time

As soon as Going-to-the-Sun Road opens in late spring, the relatively low-elevation trail to a series of spectacular falls is ready to hike and is best accessed via the interpretive Glacier Park Boat Company tour. The trail to Baring Falls is a brief 75 yards from the upper boat dock and maneuverable for strollers or people unaccustomed to hiking at elevation. The trail from the upper boat dock to Saint Mary Falls and on to Virginia Falls is a bit more challenging yet offers shade and breeze on hot or inclement-weather days.

Finding the Trail

From Rising Sun Motor Inn, cross Going-to-the-Sun Road heading south and see the BOAT TOURS sign. The large parking area offers shade for hot summer parking. Take the boat tour to Baring Falls.

Another option is to drive Going-to-the-Sun Road 3 miles west from Rising Sun Motor Inn to the Sun Point parking area. The trailhead is west of the picnic area.

A third option is 3.5 miles west of Rising Sun Motor Inn at the Sunrift Gorge pull-off, which is often quite congested—use caution here. See the

TRAIL USE
Day hiking, child-friendly
LENGTH
5.0 miles, 3–5 hours
VERTICAL FEET
±255' (±285' from Going-to-the-Sun Road)
DIFFICULTY
1 **2** 3 4 5
TRAIL TYPE
Out-and-back
SURFACE TYPE
Dirt and rock
START & END
BOAT DOCK:
N48° 41.445'
W113° 31.476'
UPPER BOAT DOCK AND TRAILHEAD:
N48° 40.525'
W113° 35.673'
SAINT MARY FALLS TRAILHEAD ON GOING-TO-THE-SUN ROAD:
N48° 40.489'
W113° 36.520'

FEATURES
Waterfalls
Flora, Wildlife
Geologic Interest

FACILITIES
Tour boat, Shuttle
Campground and store
Picnic area

163

large SAINT MARY FALLS sign; the trailhead is on the south side of Going-to-the-Sun Road.

Trail Description

The tour boat ride from Rising Sun Boat Dock aboard Glacier Park Boat Company's *Joy II* and *Little Chief* departs five times a day for an interpretive cruise up the lake to the upper boat dock at Baring Falls. The lakeshore-hugging trail from Baring Falls to Saint Mary Falls provides stunning scenes across Saint Mary Lake to 9,030-foot Citadel Mountain—if you look closely, you can see the white slash of Virginia Falls among the trees of Dusty Star Mountain, the northeast subsummit of Citadel. Almost-a-Dog Mountain at 8,922 feet and Little Chief Mountain at 9,541 feet hem the lake just south of Citadel.

The twice-daily ranger-led hike is an excellent choice and departs aboard the tour boat. The ranger's fascinating details include wildlife, flowers, and geological marvels, such as the red argillite along the trail. As the boat passes Wild Goose Island, the boat captain reveals American Indian lore: It's said that a young Indian warrior met and fell in love with a beautiful woman from another tribe, but their elders forbade that relationship. The young lovers ran away but were chased by a war party determined to

Waterfall

Wildlife

Flora

Geologic Interest

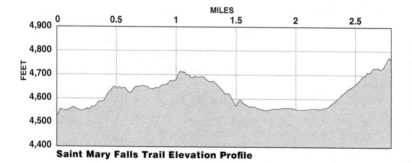

Saint Mary Falls Trail Elevation Profile

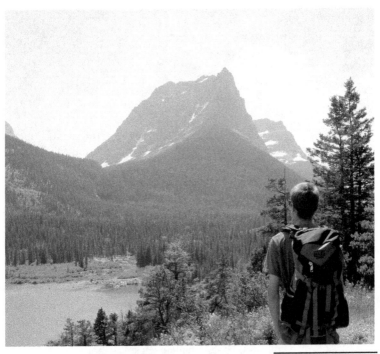

Saint Mary Falls Trail *provides dramatic viewpoints all along the trail, including Dusty Star and Citadel Mountains.*

The free park shuttle allows for parking at the Rising Sun Boat Dock, riding the tour boat and hiking to the falls and Going-to-the-Sun Road, and shuttling back to your vehicle.

bring them home. The Great Spirit took pity on the young couple and turned them into geese, forever together on Wild Goose Island. The island is actually a tower of Altyn Formation limestone based at lake bottom, some 300 feet below the boat. The ranger hikes with groups from the Baring Falls Boat Dock to Saint Mary Falls and back on the 3-mile round-trip in 3.5 hours, returning in time to catch the next boat back to Rising Sun Boat Dock.

The trail drops from Going-to-the-Sun Road down about 230 feet to lake level and traverses along and above the lakeshore to the inlet at the base of Virginia Falls. Rangers note that the leading cause of death in Glacier is drowning. The water is only a few degrees above freezing, even in late summer, and is a contributor to hypothermia and drowning. Posted signs declare DANGER: KEEP OFF the rocks at the falls. The hike climbs about 280 feet over a mile and passes a series of waterfalls of Virginia Creek.

Waterfall

Once you arrive at Virginia Falls, you can either take the footbridge over the pool at the base of the falls (and there's a pit toilet nearby), or proceed up the trail another 0.2 mile to a viewpoint. You will also see trail signs for Red Eagle Lake Trail departing east—this is a very long hike that ends either in the community of Saint Mary or at a T with a south route to Red Eagle Lake. Be prepared for a long, relatively flat trudge alongside Saint Mary Lake if you choose the Red Eagle Lake route.

🚶 MILESTONES

►1   0.0   Start from Rising Sun Boat Dock and ride the tour boat.

►2   0.0   Hike from upper boat dock.

►3   0.1   Spur trail to Baring Falls and return to boat dock.

►4   0.5   Horse cutoff trail; continue west.

►5   0.84   First junction with spur trail to Going-to-the-Sun Road; proceed left/southwest.

►6   1.28   Second junction with spur trail to Going-to-the-Sun Road; proceed left/southwest.

►7   1.29   Junction; stay left/southwest onto Saint Mary Falls Trail toward falls.

►8   1.78   Cross bridge over Saint Mary Falls.

►9   2.5   Virginia Falls. Return to boat dock.

Otokomi Lake/Rose Creek Trail

From Going-to-the-Sun Road and the Rising Sun area, it doesn't seem possible that a gentle valley hike is accessible since tall peaks encase the area; however, the valley slices between the 7,935-foot Otokomi Mountain to the east and 8,826-foot Goat Mountain to the west and provides a lovely route into the backcountry with a rewarding, trout-filled lake at the trail's terminus.

Best Time

Mid-July through October, the Otokomi Lake/Rose Creek Trail is mostly snow-free. Downed trees may inhibit travel in the first 3 miles; trail crews clear debris in July. Snow patches cover trail sections, but, in general, the route will be passable.

Finding the Trail

From the Rising Sun Motor Inn store, the trail begins on the left/north and heads east into Rose Creek drainage. The trail is also accessible from the cabin area, 50 yards from the bathhouse and along the north vehicle loop. There is a small metal trail sign and a bright-red fire hydrant behind the sign. Proceed 50 yards north on the trail to a junction, and take a hard right (east).

Trail Description

The first 2 miles are cloaked with a thick forest of Douglas fir, lodgepole pines, and an understory of wild roses, huckleberry bushes, Indian paintbrush,

TRAIL USE
Day hiking, youth-friendly

LENGTH
10.5 miles, 4–6 hours

VERTICAL FEET
±1,900'

DIFFICULTY
1 2 **3** 4 5

TRAIL TYPE
Out-and-back

SURFACE TYPE
Dirt

START & END
N48° 41.846'
W113° 31.122'

FEATURES
Flora
Geologic Interest
Historic Interest
Wildlife
Birds
Lake
Fishing
Views

FACILITIES
Campground, Cabins
Camp store
Picnic area
Bathhouse
Restrooms
Restaurant, Gift shop
Tour boat
Shuttle

167

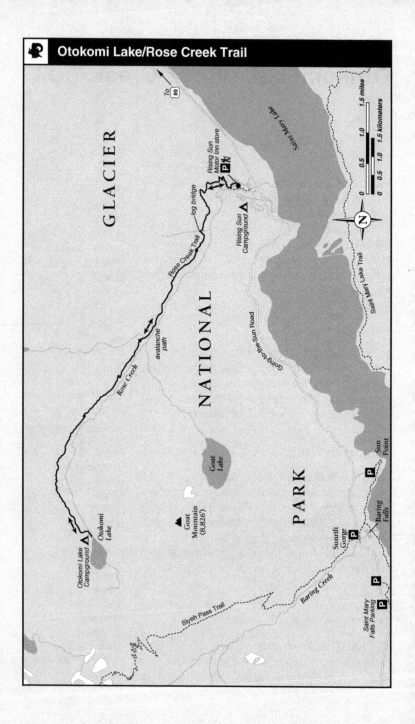

Otokomi Lake/Rose Creek Trail

To 89

GLACIER

Saint Mary Lake

Rising Sun Motor Inn store

P

Rising Sun Campground

log bridge

Rose Creek Trail

avalanche path

NATIONAL

Rose Creek

Going-to-the-Sun Road

Saint Mary Lake Trail

N

Goat Lake

Sun Point

P

PARK

Baring Falls

Goat Mountain (8,826')

Otokomi Lake Campground

Otokomi Lake

Sunrift Gorge

P

Baring Creek

P

Siyeh Pass Trail

Saint Mary Falls Parking

P

0   0.5   1.0   1.5 kilometers
0   0.5   1.0   1.5 miles

The official park signs label this Rose Creek Trail, yet local hikers, trail crew reports, and guidebooks call it Otokomi Trail.

and beargrass. At mile 2.4, an avalanche path crosses the trail from the right. Often bears will graze here, seeking winterkill in the avalanche and berries among the bushes.

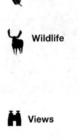 Flora

Several waterfalls loudly announce themselves along Rose Creek. Once you reach forest edge, Goat Mountain is in full and majestic view, snow-draped well into August.

Wildlife

In early July, the trail usually has four snowfield crossings, but by mid-July only two remain challenging—it's a good idea to pack a trekking pole.

Views

The final 0.5 mile is across an argillite scree slope with a view of the cirque surrounding Otokomi Lake. The trail descends about 50 feet to the foot of the lake, and here you may see large, 12- to 18-inch cutthroat trout swimming in the lake's outlet.

Geologic Interest

Three campsites, a food-hanging pole, and an outhouse are along the creek. By late July, two rocky beaches melt out on the lake's east side, although on

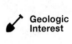 Lake

 Camping

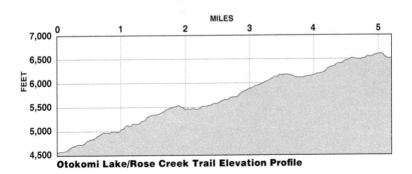

Otokomi Lake/Rose Creek Trail Elevation Profile

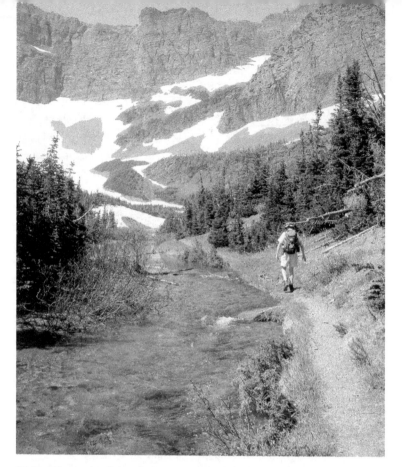

Otokomi Lake *is cradled in a high mountain cirque.*

NOTES

Otokomi, the Blackfeet word meaning "yellow fish," is the Indian name of Charlie Rose, who was the son of an American Fur Company associate. Rose Creek is most likely named for Charlie Otokomi Rose.

a hot day, these offer little shade. If you want the sun at your back, look for the rocky beach on the other side of the lake. At the mouth of the stream, you can ford the creek—it's 40°F even in mid-July. Take the thin lakeside trail to a beachlike set of rocks where you have your back to the sun for a picnic.

Upon returning to the trailhead, visit the store for cold drinks or the restaurant for an excellent meal.

Moose and bear reside here. The National Park Service recommends hiking in groups, carrying a canister of pepper spray, and making plenty of noise.

⚐ MILESTONES

▶1	0.0	Start from the Rising Sun Motor Inn store.
▶2	0.05	Optional start from cabin area parking lot
▶3	1.16	Cross a cold creek on log footbridge.
▶4	2.4	Avalanche path
▶5	5.25	Campsites, pit toilet, and lake. Return to trailhead.

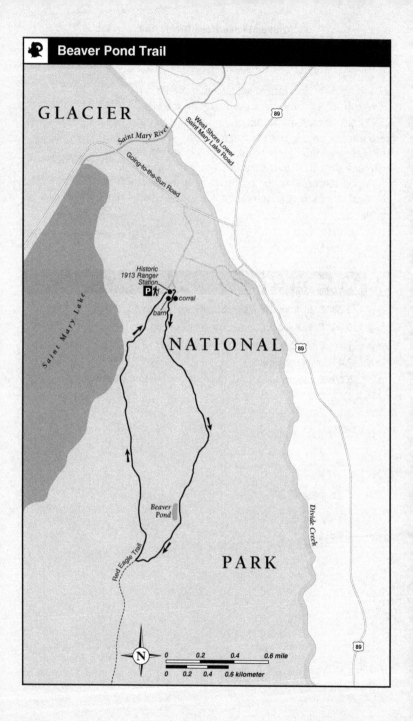

Beaver Pond Trail

GLACIER

Saint Mary River

West Shore Lower
Saint Mary Lake Road

89

Going-to-the-Sun Road

Historic
1913 Ranger
Station

P

corral

barn

NATIONAL

89

Saint Mary Lake

Beaver
Pond

Red Eagle Trail

Divide Creek

PARK

N

0   0.2   0.4   0.6 mile

0   0.2   0.4   0.6 kilometer

Beaver Pond Trail

A gentle introduction to Glacier's backcountry, Beaver Pond Trail offers exquisite views of the mountains and lake, fire ecology, wildflowers, and a century-old ranger station, perfect for first-time hikers, children, and visitors who are acclimatizing to the altitude. Additionally, the Red Eagle Lake Trail portion of the loop (beginning in a counterclockwise route) provides a wide and relatively smooth half mile, appropriate for people with mobility challenges.

Best Time

The trail is an excellent introduction to hiking and is one of the earliest trails to become snow-free, generally mid-May through late October. If the day is windy, the trail offers shelter from gusts.

Finding the Trail

From the Saint Mary Lodge at the junction of US 89 and Going-to-the-Sun Road, drive northwest on Going-to-the-Sun Road (Glacier Route 1) toward the park entrance station (do not pass through the park entrance station). At 0.25 mile, cross a small bridge and see the large brown Historic 1913 Ranger Station sign; turn left/south. Drive 0.3 mile to a large parking area. For a clockwise hike, the loop trail begins on the east edge of the parking area; walk up the grassy driveway to the Historic Ranger Station. The trailhead marker is behind the log-home structure. The loop meets Red Eagle Lake Trail to return to the parking area's southwest corner.

TRAIL USE
Day hiking, child-friendly
LENGTH
3.5 miles, 1–2 hours
VERTICAL FEET
±350'
DIFFICULTY
1 2 3 4 5
TRAIL TYPE
Loop
SURFACE TYPE
Dirt and gravel
START & END
N48° 44.315'
W113° 26.198'

FEATURES
Flora
Secluded
Geologic Interest
Historic Interest
Wildlife
Birds

FACILITIES
Ranger station
Lodging
Restaurants
Stores
Gas
Interpretive center
Campgrounds
Shuttle

Trail Description

Historic Interest

Lodgepole saplings rejuvenated the forest after the 2006 Red Eagle Fire, ignited at Red Eagle Lake; ultimately, the blaze scorched more than 32,000 acres, 19,000 of which burned the Blackfeet Indian Reservation lands.

Flora

The Historic 1913 Ranger Station at the trailhead provides a glimpse at the rugged living conditions at Glacier when it was a newly designated park. The ranger's home is a well-preserved two-story, split-log structure. Notice the axe marks—the buildings were crafted with hand tools. From the front porch, visitors can peek through windows for a view of simple furnishings. Nearby, the 1926 Lubec Barn and corral remind visitors that Glacier was a road-less region until 1932, when Going-to-the-Sun Road opened. Rangers lived in isolation, traveling on foot or horseback. The ranger station housed rangers until 1969 and was listed on the National Register of Historic Places in 1972.

The trail initially climbs through brushy cow parsnip (*Heracleum maximum*; also called Indian celery), an herb that can cause skin irritation from brushing against the leaves. American Indians made poultices from the plant to apply to bruises. The thick underbrush and woods quickly give way to wildflower-filled meadows of lupine, sticky geranium, gaillardia, and vetch. Soon, you pass through the specter of standing, dead pine trees burned in the 2006 Red Eagle Fire. Thanks to the fire, views now include the jagged skyline of the Northern Rockies.

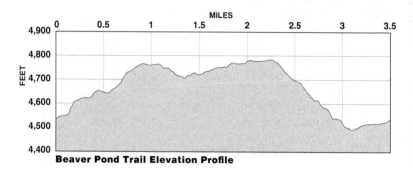

Beaver Pond Trail Elevation Profile

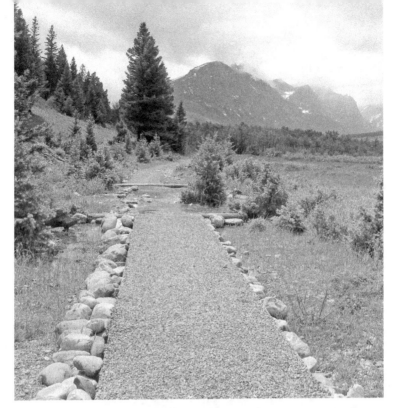

Family-friendly *Beaver Pond/Red Eagle Lake loop travels among thick wildflowers and aspens to a prairie ecosystem.*

You will see the beaver pond at 1.38 miles; the pond's access spur trail is about 100 yards ahead, and it might just be in use: moose live here, so be alert for *Alces alces* munching on willows. Frogs and birds reside here too. Look for sandpipers, red-winged blackbirds, cedar waxwings, and red-naped sapsuckers.

As you continue, notice the white geranium and larkspur, and listen for songbirds' trill. The trail meets the route to Red Eagle Lake; take the right/north route toward the trailhead and parking area. Soon, the trail approaches the shore of Saint Mary Lake, where a spur trail leads to fine picnic spots. Look toward the lake for superb photos of Red Eagle Mountain, Heavy Runner Mountain, and

Wildlife

Birds

The 1913 Historic Ranger Station and surrounding buildings were originally called the Saint Mary District, housing a ranger whose roles were protecting game from poachers, providing visitor services, and law enforcement.

other peaks surrounding the Saint Mary Valley. Often, significant winds blast past; however, keep in mind that the breezes keep mosquitoes and deerflies at bay.

MILESTONES

►1	0.0	Start from Historic 1913 Ranger Station at trailhead sign.
►2	0.08	Pass by a barn and corral.
►3	1.38	Beaver Pond
►4	1.8	Junction with Red Eagle Lake Trail; hike north on this trail toward parking lot.
►5	3.2	A side trail leads to the shore of Saint Mary Lake. Continue north on Red Eagle Lake Trail.
►6	3.5	Parking lot of Historic 1913 Ranger Station

Opposite: *Above the Siyeh Pass Trail, the high-alpine ecosystem affords little vegetation and lots of mountain views.*

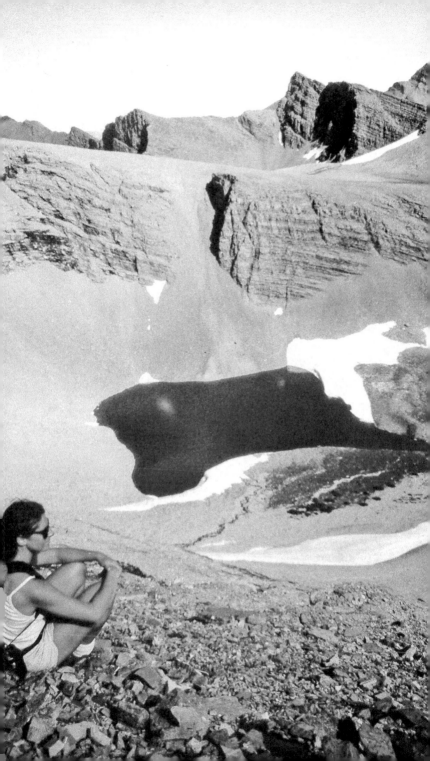

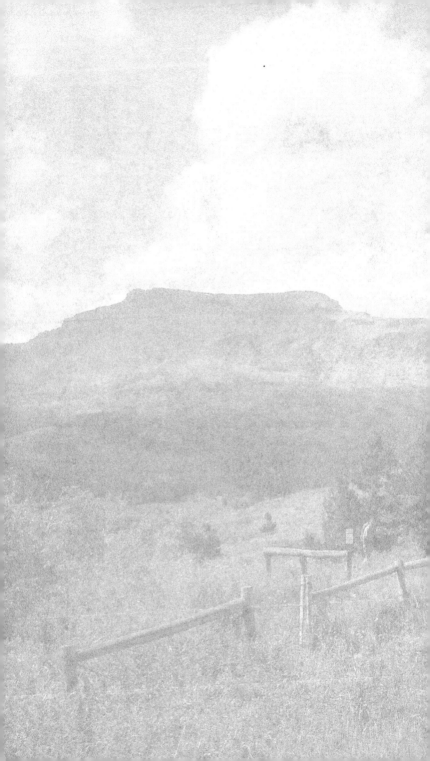

CHAPTER 3

Two Medicine and South Boundary Area

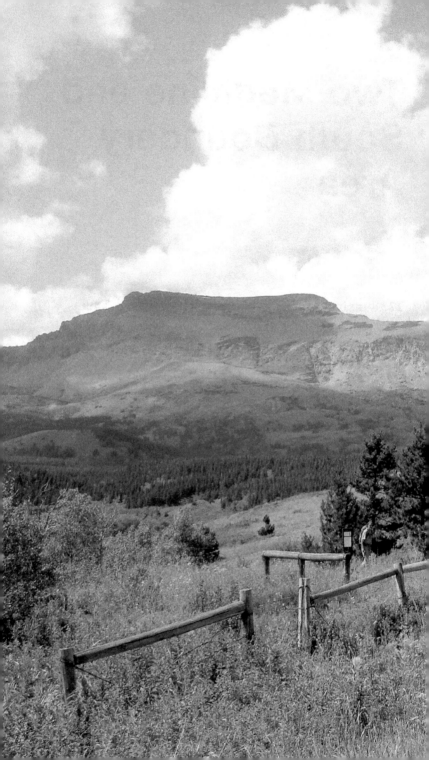

Two Medicine and South Boundary Area

Glacier's Two Medicine region stretches from the southern boundary of the park, hemmed by US 2, through East Glacier and on to Two Medicine Lake, Ranger Station, Campground, and tour boat docks via MT 49 and Two Medicine Road. Drivers must be on high alert for cattle and horses because the ranchlands here on the Blackfeet Reservation provide grasses for open-range livestock. Cattle and horses, unrestrained by fences, may be on the roadways, and it is the driver's responsibility to watch out for stock on the 1.5-million-acre Blackfeet Indian Reservation. Wildlife thrives here, too, in this remote portion of the park, prime grizzly bear habitat. Few inroads trace into the interior, yet trails zig and zag to vantage points that reveal glacier cirques and arêtes, iceberg-laden lakes, windswept peaks, and glimpses of some 9 million acres of mostly road-less area of the Rocky Mountain Front, sweeping southward to the Bob Marshall Wilderness Complex and northward into Canada. While this alpine region is lively with quaking aspens and brilliant wildflowers, it is also the only area of the park in which the Montana state flower, the pink bitterroot, survives among the rocky terrain of the Continental Divide near Marias Pass. Also of note is the pass namesake—Marias Pass was named for the Marias River, named in 1805 by Captain Meriwether Lewis for his cousin and, some speculate, his fiancée, Maria Wood. While the Corps of Discovery, the Lewis and Clark Expedition, sought this low-elevation pass over the Continental Divide, they did not find the pass and instead canoed farther up the Missouri River and southward.

Before the Going-to-the Sun Road's completion in 1932, Two Medicine was one of the busiest areas of the park, with a bustling hotel and cabins, which fell into disrepair during World War II. The few remaining buildings now house the camp store and employee quarters, leaving the campground

Opposite and overleaf: *Firebrand Pass Trail; see page 219.*

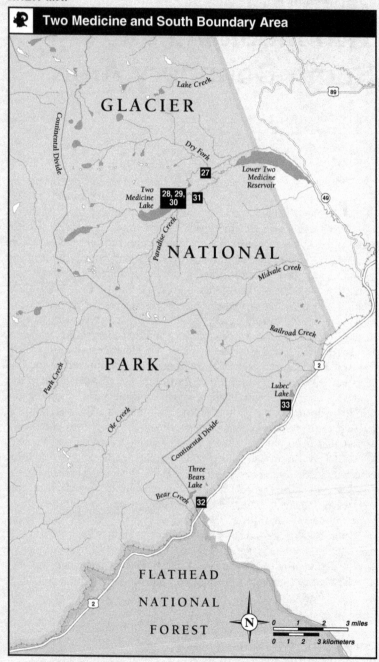

Two Medicine and South Boundary Area

GLACIER

NATIONAL

PARK

Lake Creek

Continental Divide

Dry Fork

27

Lower Two Medicine Reservoir

Two Medicine Lake

28, 29, 30 31

Paradise Creek

Midvale Creek

Railroad Creek

2

Park Creek

Ole Creek

Lubec Lake

33

Continental Divide

Three Bears Lake

Bear Creek 32

89

49

FLATHEAD

NATIONAL

FOREST

2

N

0   1   2   3 miles

0 1 2   3 kilometers

TRAIL FEATURES TABLE

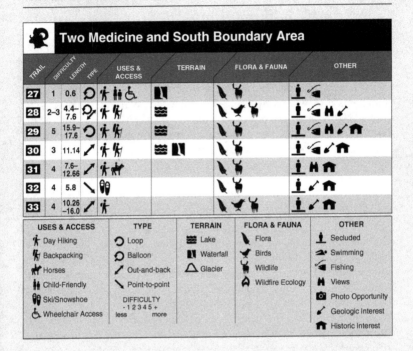

Two Medicine and South Boundary Area

TRAIL	DIFFICULTY	LENGTH	TYPE	USES & ACCESS	TERRAIN	FLORA & FAUNA	OTHER
27	1	0.6	Loop	Day Hiking, Child-Friendly, Wheelchair Access	Waterfall	Wildlife	Secluded, Fishing
28	2–3	4.4–7.6	Balloon	Day Hiking, Backpacking	Lake	Flora, Birds, Wildlife	Secluded, Fishing, Views, Geologic Interest
29	5	15.9–17.6	Loop	Day Hiking, Backpacking	Lake	Flora, Wildlife	Secluded, Fishing, Views, Geologic Interest, Historic Interest
30	3	11.14	Out-and-back	Day Hiking, Backpacking	Lake, Waterfall	Flora, Wildlife	Secluded, Fishing, Geologic Interest, Historic Interest
31	4	7.6–12.66	Out-and-back	Day Hiking, Horses		Flora, Wildlife	Secluded, Views, Historic Interest
32	4	5.8	Point-to-point	Ski/Snowshoe		Flora, Wildlife	Secluded, Geologic Interest, Historic Interest
33	4	10.26–16.0	Out-and-back	Day Hiking		Flora, Birds, Wildlife	Secluded, Geologic Interest, Historic Interest

USES & ACCESS	TYPE	TERRAIN	FLORA & FAUNA	OTHER
Day Hiking	Loop	Lake	Flora	Secluded
Backpacking	Balloon	Waterfall	Birds	Swimming
Horses	Out-and-back	Glacier	Wildlife	Fishing
Child-Friendly	Point-to-point		Wildfire Ecology	Views
Ski/Snowshoe	DIFFICULTY			Photo Opportunity
Wheelchair Access	- 1 2 3 4 5 +			Geologic Interest
	less more			Historic Interest

as the area of most activity at night—ranger-led campfire talks enthrall visitors with discourse on the flora and fauna here.

East Glacier, however, is bustling all summer long, thanks in part to the Amtrak station's twice-daily stops, and the century-old Glacier Park Lodge, with vibrant gardens, a swimming pool, a restaurant, a gift shop, and a golf course. Other eateries, mom-and-pop motels, artisans' wares, and the Glacier Gateway Outfitters' horses enliven summers. By late fall, most tourist attractions are shuttered against the intense winters of the Northern Rockies. Along US 2 is yet another historic hotel, the Izaak Walton Inn, built by the Great Northern Railway to house employees. It's now a year-round recreation center for cross-country skiing in the winter and hiking, biking, and fly-fishing the rest of the year.

Permits and Maps

No permit is required to hike inside Glacier; however, a Blackfeet Conservation/Recreation Use Permit is required for hiking, biking, horseback riding, and fishing on the reservation (call 406-338-7207 for more information). A fishing permit is not required to fish in Glacier, but a Montana fishing license is required outside the park and is for sale at most outfitters, sporting goods stores, and some grocery stores. Fishing is catch-and-release only in certain areas for cutthroat trout—check with the entrance stations or ranger stations for details. The daily catch-and-possession limit is five fish, with a maximum of two cutthroat trout, two burbot (ling), one northern pike, two mountain whitefish, five lake whitefish, five kokanee salmon, five grayling, five rainbow trout, and five lake trout. The following creeks are closed to fishing for their entire length: Ole, Park, Muir, Coal, Nyack, Fish, Lee, Otatso, Boulder, and Kennedy Creeks.

Free park maps are available at entrance stations. Each of the park's lodging properties offers rudimentary local-area maps with details of trailhead access. Excellent maps are available for purchase at the in-park bookstores, gift shops, and grocery stores, as well as through the Glacier National Park Conservancy's bookstore in the West Glacier train depot, sporting goods shops, and general stores outside the park and online.

Opposite: *Oldman Lake, along the Dawson-Pitamakan Pass Trail, hosts a campground, fishing, and plenty of wildflowers.*

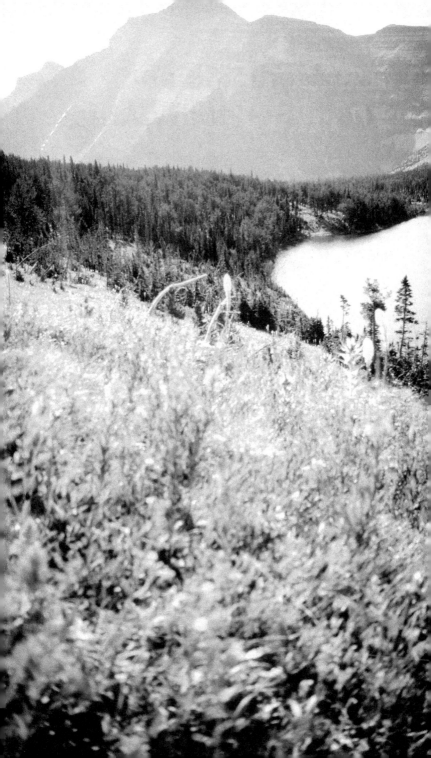

Two Medicine and South Boundary Area

Cobalt Lake via
Two Medicine Pass Trail

The ascent to Cobalt Lake climbs between Painted Tepee and Sinopah Mountains through a glaciated valley and to the top of a glacial moraine lush with wildflowers. There, snow hangs on north-facing slopes well into midsummer, and breezes splash chilled waters onto the shoreline.

TRAIL 30

Day hiking,
backpacking
11.14 miles
Out-and-back
Difficulty 1 2 **3** 4 5

Mount Henry Trail to Scenic Point

As one of the park's iconic trails, the Mount Henry Trail provides hikers with unique options to access Scenic Point. Historically, visitors rode horses on the trail, as they can today from East Glacier's Glacier Gateway Outfitters, or explorers can hike from the Two Medicine area, an arduous climb that eventually reaches treeline and finally the viewpoint.

TRAIL 31

Day hiking, horses
7.6 or 12.66 miles
Out-and-back
Difficulty 1 2 3 **4** 5

Autumn Creek Trail

Cross-country skiers and snowshoers glide into the backcountry through aspen, Douglas fir, and lodge-pole pine forest, following in the tracks of a hired guide or seasoned winter explorer, past avalanche paths and into a mountain cirque, the realm of mountain goats and blue grouse. This trail is perfect for experiencing the park's quietest season.

TRAIL 32

Cross-country skiing
5.8 miles
Point-to-point
Difficulty 1 2 3 **4** 5

Firebrand Pass Trail

Initially, the trail passes through aspen groves near a marshy meadow before quickly climbing from 5,500 to 6,951 feet in 2.4 miles above treeline, which provides views eastward over the Blackfeet Indian Reservation lands and northward deep into the park's backcountry.

TRAIL 33

Day hiking
10.26 or 16.0 miles
Out-and-back
Difficulty 1 2 3 **4** 5

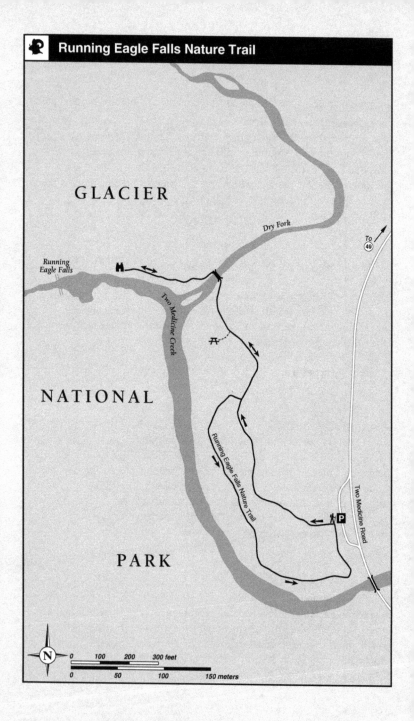

GLACIER

Dry Fork

*Running
Eagle Falls*

Two Medicine Creek

To
49

NATIONAL

Running Eagle Falls Nature Trail

Two Medicine Road

P

PARK

N

| 0 | 100 | 200 | 300 feet |

| 0 | 50 | 100 | 150 meters |

Running Eagle Falls Nature Trail (aka Trick Falls)

The trail is wide, mostly flat, and wheelchair-accessible (unless exceedingly muddy) until the narrow wooden footbridge over Two Medicine River. Note that the bridge is removed and reinstalled annually to avoid damage from ice and high water; if the bridge is not in place, the hike still reveals the spectacular Running Eagle Falls as it roars over a cliff and through a cave. The double falls is visible from the riverside at the confluence of the Dry Fork and Two Medicine River. The background is impressive and camera-worthy, with 9,513-foot Rising Wolf Mountain to the northwest and 7,831-foot Spot Mountain to the northeast.

Best Time

As soon as the road opens, May through October, the brief but rewarding walk from Two Medicine Road meanders through a forest of pines and black cottonwood trees. When other trails are windy, Running Eagle tends to be protected from the strongest gusts.

Finding the Trail

The trailhead is 1.8 miles west of the park entrance station on the north side of Two Medicine Road. The parking lot is well marked with a sign for Running Eagle Falls (Trick Falls). The trail begins at the middle of the parking lot lanes, just north of two large signs, and heads northwest past a small metal signpost. The trail wraps back to the southwest edge of the parking area on pavement.

TRAIL USE
Day hiking, child-friendly, wheelchair accessible

LENGTH
0.6 mile, 30 minutes–1 hour

VERTICAL FEET
±42'

DIFFICULTY
1 2 3 4 5

TRAIL TYPE
Balloon

SURFACE TYPE
Pavement, gravel, and dirt

START & END
N48° 29.765'
W113° 20.896'

FEATURES
Waterfall
Flora
Secluded
Wildlife
Fishing

FACILITIES
Pit toilet
Picnic area
Campground
Camp store
Ranger station

Trial Description

Flora

As you drive toward
the park's Two
Medicine Entrance
Station, look out
for cattle herds and
horses on the road—
this is open range on
the 1.5-million-acre
Blackfeet Indian
Reservation: animals
graze and move
about unrestrained by
fences.

Waterfall

Running Eagle Falls Nature Trail initially rambles
through fir and spruce forest to a riparian area
with some brushy sections and wildflower spots
of arnica, sticky geranium, thimbleberry, western
mountain ash, and yellow salsify, also called goats-
beard. The park's small placards identify plants,
such as the black cottonwood trees, ancient natives.
The seeds need very moist soil to germinate and are
often found along rivers that flood annually—Dry
Creek is a prime example of spring scouring washouts and summer dry-ups.

The final reward is the stacked double waterfalls. The falls are nicknamed Trick Falls because
of the double falls. In 1981, the falls were renamed
from Trick Falls to Running Eagle Falls for an
1800s Blackfeet woman warrior whose vision quest
took place in the area. Her Blackfeet name was
Pitamakan.

You might hear the 40-foot cataract before
you see it as the water from Two Medicine Creek
surges down to meet Dry Creek. During spring
runoff, it's difficult to detect the lower falls, but
by midsummer, the upper fall recedes enough
to detail the lower fall, separated by rock. In late
summer, the upper fall dries up, revealing the
grotto where the lower fall gushes.

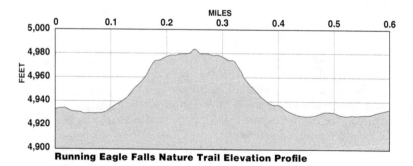

Running Eagle Falls Nature Trail Elevation Profile

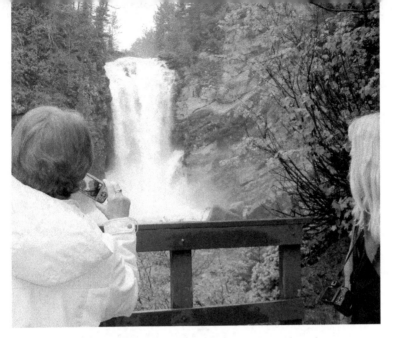

Running Eagle Falls Trail *is one of the few wheelchair-accessible trails in Glacier.*

The trail proceeds downriver to the footbridge, which then threads up to the base of the falls. The cascading water pools into a frothy emerald green to turquoise blue, depending upon the sky and light. Return via the footbridge; then take the right fork at the sign and follow the trail as it wends back to the parking lot.

🚶	**MILESTONES**	
▶1	0.0	Start from the Two Medicine roadside pull-off at the Running Eagle Falls Trailhead.
▶2	0.01	Follow the trail straight north.
▶3	0.2	Footbridge
▶4	0.26	Viewpoint
▶5	0.31	Falls
▶6	0.41	Return via loop trail to the west.
▶7	0.6	Trail reaches the parking lot at the west end of the parking spaces.

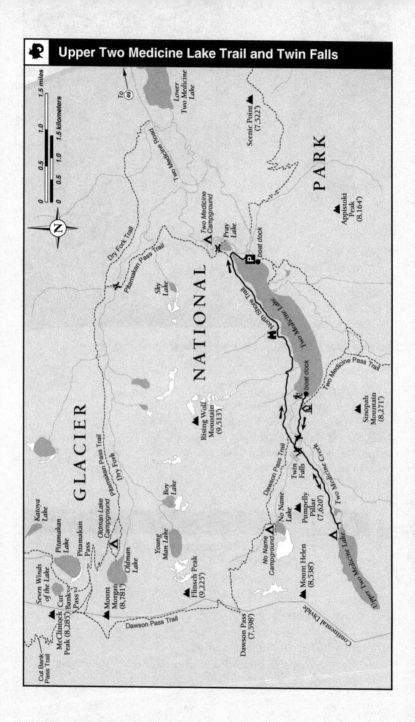

Upper Two Medicine Lake Trail and Twin Falls

Lower Two Medicine Lake

Scenic Point (7,522')

PARK

Appistoki Peak (8,164')

Two Medicine Road

Dry Fork Trail

Pitamakan Pass Trail

Sky Lake

Two Medicine Campground

Pray Lake

boat dock

P

North Shore Trail

Two Medicine Lake

NATIONAL

Rising Wolf Mountain (9,513')

boat dock

Two Medicine Pass Trail

Sinopah Mountain (8,271')

GLACIER

Oldman Lake Campground

Pitamakan Pass Trail

Dry Fork

Boy Lake

Dawson Pass Trail

Twin Falls

Katoya Lake

Pitamakan Lake

Pitamakan Pass

Oldman Lake

Young Man Lake

Flinsch Peak (9,225')

No Name Lake

Pumpelly Pillar (7,620')

Two Medicine Creek

Seven Winds of the Lake

McClintock Peak (8,285')

Cut Bank Pass

Mount Morgan (8,781')

No Name Campground

Mount Helen (8,538')

Upper Two Medicine Lake

Cut Bank Pass Trail

Dawson Pass Trail

Dawson Pass (7,598')

Continental Divide

Upper Two Medicine Lake Trail and Twin Falls

From Upper Two Medicine Lake, impressive 7,600- to 9,000-foot peaks appear to rise directly from the 40°F water—which by winter is sealed under several feet of lake ice. On the immediate horizon from the beach is, left to right (south to north), Two Medicine Peak, Mount Ellsworth, Never Laughs Mountain, Painted Tepee Mountain, Mount Sinopah, Mount Rockwell, Lone Walker Mountain, Pumpelly Pillar, and Mount Helen. It's into these sentries that this trail climbs.

Best Time

Beginning in mid-June, when ice recedes from Two Medicine Lake, the trail will most likely be snow-free, except for the final approach to Upper Two Medicine Lake. The best hiking is through early October. Because the legendary winds stir up afternoons, morning hikes are usually calmer.

Finding the Trail

From the historic 1913 Two Medicine Camp Store, walk the shoreline south to the Glacier Park Boat Company's dock, and book a trip aboard the *Sinopah*—several trips depart daily from early June to early September. The trailhead begins at the western boat dock. Another option is to access it via the Dawson Pass Trail that follows the lake's northern shore and begins at the Two Medicine Campground.

TRAIL USE
Day hiking, backpacking

LENGTH
7.6 miles (balloon) or 4.4 miles (out-and-back with boat ride), 3–6 hours

VERTICAL FEET
±413'

DIFFICULTY
1 **2 3** 4 5

TRAIL TYPE
Balloon or out-and-back

SURFACE TYPE
Dirt

START & END
EASTERN BOAT DOCK:
N48° 29.020'
W113° 22.185'
TRAILHEAD AT WESTERN
BOAT DOCK:
N48° 28.458'
W113° 24.531'

FEATURES
Lake, Fishing
Flora
Geologic Interest
Wildlife
Birds
Views

FACILITIES
Ranger station
Campground and store
Boat dock, Tour boat
Canoe rentals

Trail Description

For an educational and fun interpretive trip, take the Glacier Park Boat Company tour on the *Sinopah,* a 45-foot wooden tour boat, from the Two Medicine Boat Dock across the lake to the western boat dock. Here, the trailhead to Upper Two Medicine Lake and its backcountry campground leads west. The boat company offers a free backcountry 0.9-mile hike to Twin Falls, also departing along the Upper Two Medicine Lake Trail.

A few steps past the junction to Twin Falls, yet on the Upper Two Medicine Trail, look west for a photogenic view of Pumpelly Pillar, a 7,620-foot-tall, glacially carved, cone-shaped peak. It was named for a railway survey party leader who traveled this area in 1883. Trees soon thin as you access higher elevations. Wildflower meadows host glacier lilies, lupine, Indian paintbrush, and thimbleberries.

Along the way, the trail passes above a small lake, which attracts waterfowl, such as Canada geese and mallards, but the real lake is just 0.25 mile farther—a rewarding climb next to a rumbling falls. Even in late June, ice borders Upper Two Medicine Lake like brocade lace. The dominant peak at the lake's western shore is Lone Walker Mountain, part of the Continental Divide. Four

Views

Flora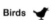

Birds

Lake

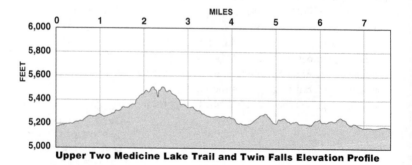

Upper Two Medicine Lake Trail and Twin Falls Elevation Profile

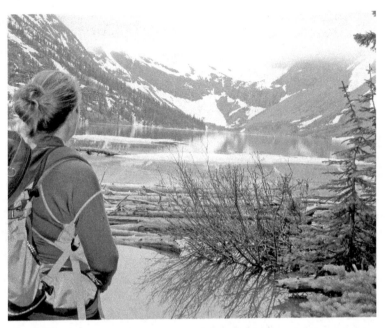

Upper Two Medicine Lake's *name is derived from an intended medicine lodge ceremony between the Blackfeet and Blood Indians.*

backcountry campsites (with a pit toilet) offer lake and mountain views. Notice the red argillite walls, remnants of a shallow inland sea. The Precambrian Belt Series sedimentary rock is 1,600 million to 800 million years old.

If you return along the same route, consider taking the Twin Falls spur trail, a 15-minute side trip to a double falls. Also consider extending your hike to venture along Two Medicine Lake's northern edge via the Dawson Pass Trail to the parking lot, campground, camp store, and boat dock at Two Medicine. As you near the campground, remain on the main trail—the footpaths departing here are wildlife trails and a fishermen's spot. The trail leads to a footbridge and into the campground.

 Camping

 Geologic Interest

MILESTONES

▶1	0.0	Start from Two Medicine Boat Dock and ride the *Sinopah*.
▶2	0.0	Disembark at the western dock and see the trailhead sign a few steps ashore.
▶3	0.17	Junction with Two Medicine Pass Trail; hike west. Outhouse is on your left.
▶4	0.7	Junction with Dawson Cutoff Trail; continue straight/west.
▶5	0.9	Junction with spur trail to Twin Falls
▶6	1.0	Twin Falls
▶7	2.3	Upper Two Medicine Lake
▶8	3.7	Return to Dawson Cutoff Trail junction and head northeast.
▶9	3.88	Take Dawson Pass Trail east along the northern edge of Two Medicine Lake.
▶10	6.7	Spur trail to lake
▶11	6.88	Junction with Pitamakan Pass Trail; keep right/east.
▶12	6.92	Footbridge over Two Medicine River and Campground
▶13	7.1	Camp store and parking area
▶14	7.6	Two Medicine Boat Dock

NOTES

Like many of Glacier's trails, the routes in the Two Medicine area served horseback travelers who had arrived by train and stayed in rustic chalets, each a day's trail ride apart, or in canvas tents and tepees. Today's camp store is the Two Medicine Chalet's dining hall, from which, in 1930, President Herbert Hoover declared the chalet the Summer White House.

Dawson Pass and Pitamakan Pass Trail (Oldman Lake)

Two mountain passes, four crystalline lakes with campsites, dozens of snow-encrusted peaks, and meadow after meadow of wildflowers make the arduous Dawson and Pitamakan Passes among the finest routes in the park. The 17.6-mile trail can be abbreviated by taking the Glacier Park Boat Company's *Sinopah* across Two Medicine Lake, a tour that is most worthy for the interpretive session and the glimpse into the depths of an extraordinarily clear mountain lake. Native trout are visible as the historic boat motors across the 2.5-mile-long lake. Nine peaks etch the skyline.

Best Time

The trail is clear of snow and downed trees by mid-July and remains passable through early October. Earlier summer promises a buggy hike. Early fall might provide fresh snow.

Finding the Trail

From the historic 1913 Two Medicine Camp Store, walk the shoreline south to the Glacier Park Boat Company's dock, and book a tour aboard the *Sinopah* across Two Medicine Lake—several trips depart daily from early June to early September. Trailhead begins at the western boat dock.

Trail Description

The loop can be hiked in either direction; however, this clockwise description leads west via the tour

---

TRAIL USE
Day hiking, backpacking

LENGTH
15.9 miles (including tour boat shuttle) or 17.6 miles; 12–18 hours or 2-day backpack

VERTICAL FEET
+3,460'/–3,477'

DIFFICULTY
1 2 3 4 **5**

TRAIL TYPE
Loop

SURFACE TYPE
Boardwalk, dirt, and gravel

START & END
EASTERN BOAT DOCK:
N48° 29.020'
W113° 22.185'
WITHOUT BOAT RIDE:
N48° 29.411'
W113° 21.826'

FEATURES
Flora
Geologic Interest
Historic Interest
Wildlife, Views
Lake, Fishing

FACILITIES
Ranger station
Gas
Boat tour, Canoe rentals
Campgrounds and store

197

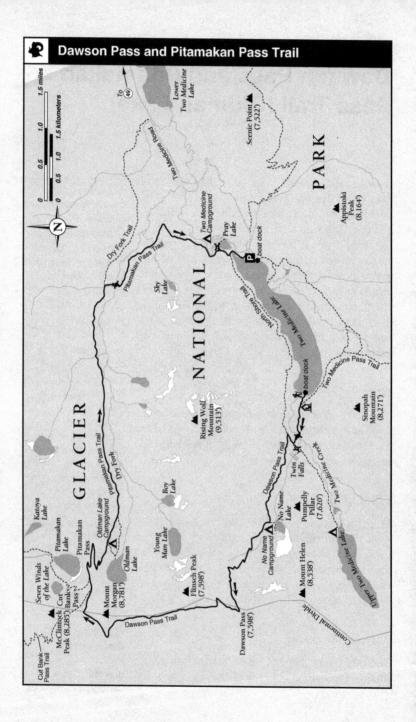

Dawson Pass and Pitamakan Pass Trail

To (49)

Lower Two Medicine Lake

Scenic Point (7,522')

P A R K

Appistoki Peak (8,164')

Two Medicine Road

Dry Fork Trail

Pitamakan Pass Trail

Sky Lake

Two Medicine Campground

Pray Lake

boat dock

N A T I O N A L

North Shore Trail

Two Medicine Lake

Two Medicine Pass Trail

Sinopah Mountain (8,271')

boat dock

Rising Wolf Mountain (9,513')

G L A C I E R

Katoya Lake

Pitamakan Lake

Pitamakan Pass

Oldman Lake Campground

Dry Fork

Pitamakan Pass Trail

Boy Lake

Dawson Pass Trail

Twin Falls

Two Medicine Creek

Seven Winds of the Lake

McClintock Peak (8,285')

Cut Bank Pass

Mount Morgan (8,781')

Oldman Lake

Young Man Lake

Flinsch Peak (7,598')

No Name Lake

Pumpelly Pillar (7,620')

No Name Campground

Upper Two Medicine Lake

Cut Bank Pass Trail

Dawson Pass Trail

Mount Helen (8,538')

Dawson Pass (7,598')

Continental Divide

1.5 miles
1.5 kilometers
1.0
0.5
0

boat to Dawson Pass first. From the lake's middle, Dawson Pass is visible in a saddle to the west.

From the western dock, the trail initially cruises through a buggy, damp area replete with ferns and thimbleberries but soon feels more arid as it climbs among pine and spruce trees. Pay attention to several trail junctions, all clearly marked as you move from the boat dock to Dawson Pass Trailhead. From here, it's uphill to the 7,600-foot pass. En route, the 12-acre No Name Lake, at 2.3 miles from the boat dock, provides a scenic lunch spot or campsite—reservations required. Take a 0.1-mile spur trail to reach three campsites and a pit toilet near the lakeshore.

The trail passes through Bighorn Basin, a bowl of wildflowers, as it climbs 1,650 more feet to the pass. Carved by glacial action during the last ice age, the basin lives up to its name. Bighorn sheep, *Ovis canadensis*, graze the shoulder of Rising Wolf Mountain.

At 4.2 miles and 7,600 feet elevation, Dawson Pass's rock cairn reveals new views of Two Medicine Lake, Mount Henry, and peaks of the Lewis Range. Dominating the western view is 9,494-foot Mount Phillips and remnants of Lupfer Glacier about 3,000 feet below Phillips's summit.

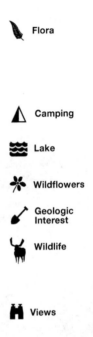

Flora

Camping

Lake

Wildflowers

Geologic Interest

Wildlife

Views

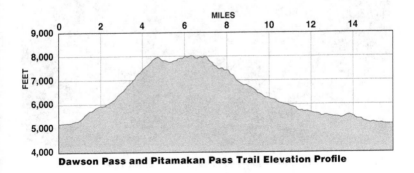

Dawson Pass and Pitamakan Pass Trail Elevation Profile

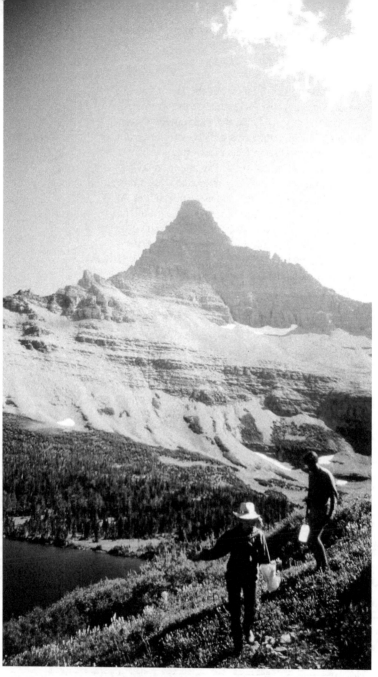

Oldman Lake, *on a spur off the Dawson-Pitamakan Pass Trail, has a campground with views.*

Another option that adds 3.8 miles is to access the Pitamakan Pass Trailhead via the Two Medicine Campground Loop A. Cross the river on the footbridge. The trail sign indicates the route to Oldman Lake and North Shore Trail. Hike 0.1 mile to the junction with the Dawson Pass Trail on the right/west; to the left/east is Pitamakan Pass Trail. Take the right trail to Dawson Pass, which follows Two Medicine Lake's northern shore.

The pass is in the saddle between 8,538-foot Mount Helen and 9,225-foot Flinsch Peak. Be prepared for strong winds scouring the alpine landscape. Only low-lying plants survive the harsh environment. The trail traverses north past Mount Morgan, allows for outstanding views at the Pitamakan Overlook, and then curves east toward Pitamakan Pass. The Cut Bank Pass junction departs left/north, and soon another junction with Pitamakan Pass Trail leads again north past Pitamakan Lake toward Cut Bank Ranger Station, but continue east and up to Pitamakan Pass.

Blackfeet Indians had vision quests in the Two Medicine Lake area, long considered a most sacred place for the Blackfeet Nation.

After the steep descent from Pitamakan Pass, the spur trail loops to Oldman Lake, a fantastic camp with a pit toilet and four tent sites—reservations required. Oldman Lake is well known for large cutthroat trout, which feed on insects; use bug repellent so you'll have time for taking photos of Flinsch Peak and Rising Wolf Mountain above the lake.

 Camping

 Lake

From Oldman Lake, the east route is gentle and generally downhill; it's also popular with grizzly bears that favor the trailside huckleberries. The rest of the route down Dry Fork cruises through an open pine forest replete with beargrass and wildflowers. The trail turns south at a junction with Dry Fork Trail. Remain on the Pitamakan Pass Trail, which is also the Continental Divide Trail.

 Wildlife

 Wildflowers

 Lake

The trail ends at the bridge over Two Medicine River, immediately below the petite Pray Lake at the Two Medicine Campground.

 Camping

▶1   0.0   Start from Two Medicine Boat Dock and ride the *Sinopah*.

▶2   0.0   Disembark at the western dock and see the trailhead sign a few steps ashore.

▶3   0.17   Junction with Two Medicine Pass Trail; hike straight/west. Outhouse is on your left.

▶4   0.7   Junction with Dawson Cutoff Trail. Hike right/north to Dawson Pass.

▶5   0.87   Junction with Dawson Pass Trail; turn left/west.

▶6   2.34   Junction with No Name Lake

▶7   4.2   Dawson Pass

▶8   7.2   Junction with Cut Bank Pass Trail; stay right/east for Pitamakan Pass.

▶9   7.37   Junction with Pitamakan Pass Trail; hike east for Pitamakan Pass.

▶10   7.58   Pitamakan Pass

▶11   8.85   Spur trail to Oldman Lake and loop

▶12   9.2   Lower spur to Oldman Lake

▶13   12.5   Junction with Dry Fork Trail; turn right/south on Pitamakan Pass Trail toward Two Medicine Campground.

▶14   12.7   Footbridge over Dry Fork Creek

▶15   14.9   Junction with Dawson Pass Trail; turn left/east.

▶16   15.0   Footbridge over Two Medicine River and Campground

▶17   15.9   Two Medicine Boat Dock

NOTES

Pitamakan was a Blackfeet Indian woman who was honored with the male name Pitawmahkn, meaning Running Eagle. A warrior, she led successful war parties until she was killed in her last raid at Flathead Lake.

Cobalt Lake via Two Medicine Pass Trail

A scenic trail with options to abbreviate the hike on both ends, the hike, on a wildflower-lined path, passes marshes, meadows, streams, a hanging bridge, waterfalls, and jagged peaks, ending at a cobalt-blue loch. The Two Medicine area in general has fewer backcountry visitors than the other east-of-the-Continental-Divide areas, perhaps because there is no longer chalet lodging. The Two Medicine Campground often fills with local campers and a few travelers who've heard about the scenic lake, trails, and peaks. Glacier Park Boat Company's *Sinopah* provides backcountry access via the upper Two Medicine Boat Dock, which can be buggy, and shortens the hike to Cobalt Lake, although tour-boat passengers/hikers will miss a series of ponds where great blue herons, moose, and beavers reside. See the sidebar on page 207 for the shorter 8.8-mile option.

Best Time

Vibrant wildflowers line the trail when snow melts, from early July through early October. The tour boat runs daily mid-June to early September and eliminates 1.3 miles each way to Cobalt Lake—check locally for daily departure times.

Finding the Trail

From the Two Medicine Lake Boat Dock, see the trailhead sign immediately south of the Glacier Park Boat Company ticket booth, between the booth and the lake. The sign reads TWO MEDICINE SOUTH SHORE TRAIL and lists several overlooks, viewpoints, passes, and lakes.

TRAIL USE
Day hiking, backpacking
LENGTH
11.14 miles, 5–8 hours
VERTICAL FEET
±1,400'
DIFFICULTY
1 2 **3** 4 5
TRAIL TYPE
Out-and-back
SURFACE TYPE
Dirt, gravel, and rock
START & END
UPPER/EASTERN BOAT
DOCK: N48° 29.020'
W113° 22.185'
LOWER/WESTERN BOAT
DOCK: N48° 28.274'
W113° 24.318'

FEATURES
Flora, Secluded
Geologic Interest
Historic Interest
Wildlife, Waterfalls
Lakes, Fishing

FACILITIES
Ranger station
Stores
Interpretive center
Campgrounds
Pit toilet
Campfire program
Ranger-led hike
Tour-boat shuttle

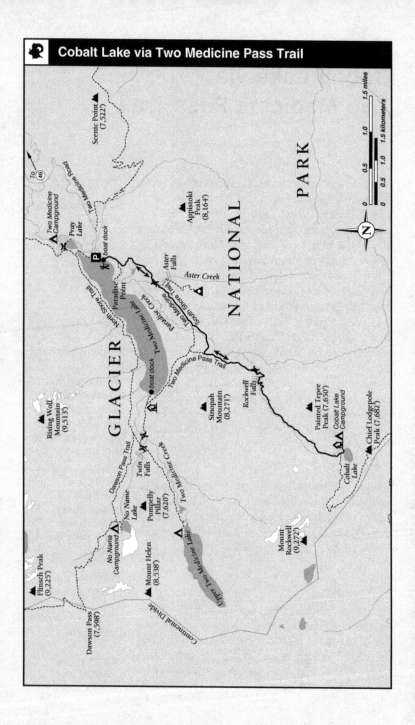

Cobalt Lake via Two Medicine Pass Trail

Scenic Point
(7,522)

To
49

Two Medicine Campground

Pray Lake

boat dock

P

Paradise Point

North Shore Trail

Aster Falls

Aster Creek

South Shore Trail

Appistoki Peak
(8,164)

N A T I O N A L

Paradise Creek

Two Medicine Creek

Two Medicine Pass Trail

G L A C I E R

Rising Wolf Mountain
(9,513)

boat dock

Sinopah Mountain
(8,271)

Rockwell Falls

Painted Tepee Peak (7,650)

Cobalt Lake Campground

Chief Lodgepole Peak (7,682)

Cobalt Lake

Dawson Pass Trail

Twin Falls

No Name Lake

Pumpelly Pillar
(7,620)

Mount Helen
(8,538)

Upper Two Medicine Lake

Mount Rockwell
(9,272)

No Name Campground

Flinsch Peak
(9,225)

Dawson Pass
(7,598)

Continental Divide

P A R K

N

1.5 miles
1.5 kilometers

0   0.5   1.0
0   0.5   1.0   1.5

Trail Description

The longer 5.57-mile route to Cobalt Lake follows the Two Medicine South Shore Trail (a somewhat deceiving name since the trail parallels but isn't near the shore), past a series of marshy potholes where waterfowl reside. Be on the lookout for moose here too. The trail has several spur routes, including a jaunt to Paradise Point, a beach on Two Medicine Lake, and another side-trip climb to Aster Falls and Aster Park Overlook, which live up to the lavender moniker.

 Wildlife

The shorter route from the upper boat dock also follows the South Shore Trail for 1.3 miles; both hiking choices meet at the junction with Two Medicine Pass Trail. The route crosses a large avalanche path where crushing snows zipped off Sinopah Mountain's ridge, leaving broken trees and excellent mountain views of the citadel-like, 8,271-foot peak in its wake.

Soon you'll hear Rockwell Falls as you approach the popular picnic spot. Many hikers turn around here, but the next 2.4 miles to Cobalt Lake are worth the switchback climb through huckleberries—make plenty of noise here in bear country. The ascent between Painted Tepee and Sinopah Mountains through a glaciated valley climbs to the top of a moraine lush with red monkeyflower, yellow

 Waterfall

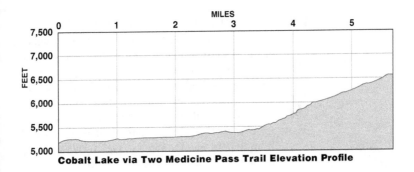

Cobalt Lake via Two Medicine Pass Trail Elevation Profile

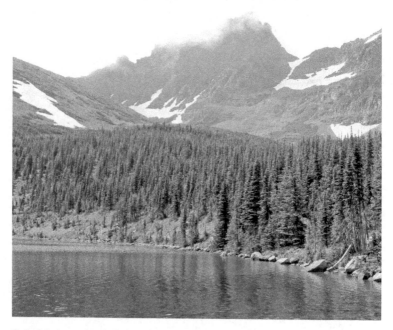

Cobalt Lake *is often the terminus—and a fine picnic spot—for summertime ranger-led hikes.*

Flora

monkeyflower, and fireweed. The trail peaks at 6,600 feet elevation. A final junction heads left and down to the lake; the right route leads up to Two Medicine Pass, Lake Isabel, and the 29-mile route on Park Creek Trail, exiting at Walton Ranger Station at Essex, Montana, a three-day backpack trip (permits required).

Lake

Chief Lodgepole Peak surrounds Cobalt Lake. Look across and above the lake to several patches of snow and you might see a grizzly bear cooling off on a bench of snow. The campground has three tent sites, a food area, and an outhouse. Beware of the massive marmot that lives under—yes, under—the outhouse. He's been known to startle many a hiker. If the outhouse door is not latched from the outside, the marmot goes inside to sit on the seat—another heart-stopping surprise.

Camping

Wildlife

🚶	**MILESTONES**	

▶1   0.0   Start from the Two Medicine Lake Boat Dock at the trail sign that reads TWO MEDICINE SOUTH SHORE TRAIL and lists several destinations, including Cobalt Lake.

▶2   1.0   Junction with Paradise Point Trail

▶3   1.16   Junction with Aster Park Overlook Trail

▶4   1.9   Junction with Two Medicine Pass Trail and trail to Two Medicine Lake's upper boat dock; stay left/south toward Cobalt Lake.

▶5   2.42   Another junction with the trail to Two Medicine Lake's upper boat dock. Stay left toward Cobalt Lake; take the left/south route.

▶6   3.28   Bridge over Rockwell Falls

▶7   5.51   Junction; Cobalt Lake to the left and Two Medicine Pass to the right

▶8   5.57   Cobalt Lake. Return to trailhead.

▶9   5.59   Cobalt Lake Campground

OPTIONS

Shorten the hike by 1.3 miles each way by riding the *Sinopah* tour boat (fee applies). From Two Medicine Lake's upper boat dock, depart the *Sinopah*, heading west along the boardwalk for 0.2 mile. See the pit toilet and trail junction sign for the Two Medicine South Shore Trail and Two Medicine Pass/Cobalt Lake, and turn left/south to follow the trail around the southwest shore of Two Medicine Lake; the trail meets the Two Medicine Pass Trail in 1.1 miles.

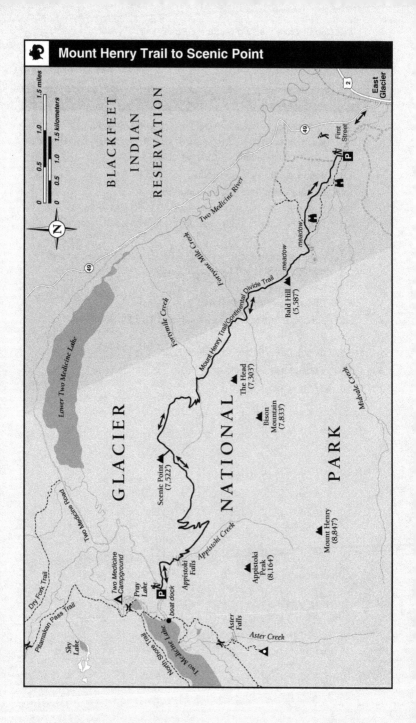

Mount Henry Trail to Scenic Point

1.5 miles

1.0

0.5

0

1.5 kilometers

1.0

0.5

0

N

BLACKFEET INDIAN RESERVATION

Two Medicine River

Fortymile Creek

Fortymile Creek

Mount Henry Trail/Continental Divide Trail

GLACIER

NATIONAL

PARK

Midvale Creek

East Glacier

2

49

First Street

P

meadow

meadow

Bald Hill (5,587')

The Head (7,303')

Bison Mountain (7,833')

Scenic Point (7,522')

Mount Henry (8,847')

Appistoki Creek

Appistoki Falls

Appistoki Peak (8,164')

Lower Two Medicine Lake

49

Two Medicine Road

Dry Fork Trail

Pitamakan Pass Trail

Sky Lake

Two Medicine Campground

Pray Lake

P

boat dock

North Shore Trail

Two Medicine Lake

Aster Falls

Aster Creek

Mount Henry Trail to Scenic Point

The Mount Henry Trail visits two separate valleys and provides scenes of different ecological systems at the eastern edge of the Rockies, called the Rocky Mountain Front. Mount Henry dominates the view to the west, and the Sweet Grass Hills pop out of the prairie some 180 miles to the east. More immediate views include Looking Glass Mountain; the Two Medicine Valley; and the glorious, aspen-thick Blackfeet Reservation's valleys, plains, and mountains, which the Indians called The Backbone of the World.

Best Time

As soon as snow melts from trails, usually early to mid-June through October, Mount Henry/Scenic Point Trail accesses several vantage points. On hot days, hike or ride early, as much of the trail is exposed to heat and wind.

Finding the Trail

From Two Medicine Road, the trailhead is 0.2 mile east of the campground junction. A large parking area on the south side of Two Medicine Road provides trailheads for Mount Henry/Scenic Point as well as Appistoki Falls. See the signpost on the east side of the parking area.

From Glacier Park Lodge in East Glacier, head north on MT 49/Looking Glass Hill Road 0.28 mile, turn west on First Street at Mountain Pine Motel, and continue 0.4 mile on a gravel road (road cuts through golf course) to the trailhead on the north side of the road.

TRAIL USE
Day hiking, horses
LENGTH
7.6 miles (from Two Medicine) or
12.66 miles (from East Glacier), 5–6 hours
VERTICAL FEET
±1,409'
DIFFICULTY
1 2 3 **4** 5
TRAIL TYPE
Out-and-back
SURFACE TYPE
Dirt
START & END
MOUNT HENRY:
N48° 29.108'
W113° 21.691'
EAST GLACIER:
N48° 26.946'
W113° 14.097'

FEATURES
Flora, Historic Interest
Wildlife, Views
FACILITIES
Lodging, Restaurants,
 Amtrak (in East Glacier)
Horse outfitters
Ranger station
 (Two Medicine)
Campground, Store
Boat dock, Rentals
Tour boat

The Blackfeet Nation's tribal headquarters is in Browning. The 1.5-million-acre Blackfeet Indian Reservation is home to about 10,000 residents, including 7,000 of the 15,560 enrolled Blackfeet tribal members.

Before World War II, hikers would find a large bell hung at the summit of Mount Henry for the hikers to ring.

Views

Flora

Trail Description

From Two Medicine Valley, the trail begins with a gentle half mile through aspens before the climb begins. En route, the noisy, picturesque Appistoki Falls is just west of the trail. At 5,600 feet elevation, the trail's first switchback ensures new vistas every few minutes, from Mount Henry to Two Medicine and Rising Wolf Mountains, and because the trail is now primarily above the treeline, it's easy to get the layout of this glaciated land. Locals call the ancient, dead trees ghost trees. These are limber pines that have succumbed to the extreme conditions: 50-mile-per-hour winds, blasting blizzards, and bone-dry summers. Yet a closer look reveals spectacular lichen and brilliant yellow flowers called stonecrop, or *Sedum lanceolatum,* which seemingly grow right out of the rock.

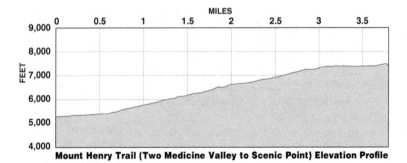

Mount Henry Trail (Two Medicine Valley to Scenic Point) Elevation Profile

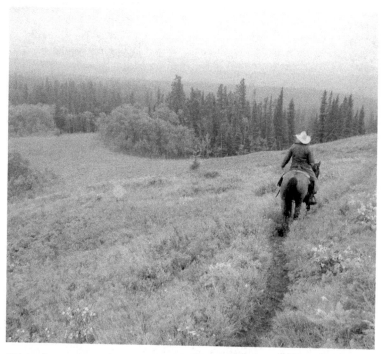

Glacier Gateway Outfitters' *Blackfeet Indian guide provides Native American interpretive information along the route up Mount Henry Trail.*

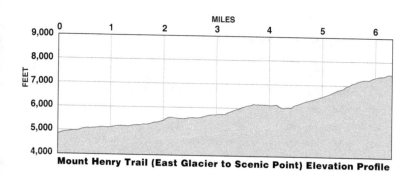

Mount Henry Trail (East Glacier to Scenic Point) Elevation Profile

The other route, a climb from East Glacier to Scenic Point, begins near Glacier Park Lodge. The route wends through the Blackfeet Indian Reservation, which borders the park's eastern boundary and is also the Continental Divide Trail. A $25 tribal recreational use permit is required and can be purchased at local shops and tourism outlets. A gravel road to the trailhead crosses through the East Glacier Golf Course, the oldest grass-greens course in Montana. From the trailhead, the route ascends into aspen groves, a patchwork of wildflowers, and pine forest to high alpine meadows at the treeline.

MILESTONES

Two Medicine Valley to Scenic Point

▶1   0.0   Start from Two Medicine Valley at the parking lot trailhead.

▶2   0.63   Spur trail leads 100 yards to Appistoki Falls overlook.

▶3   0.82   The first of eight switchbacks climbs above the treeline.

▶4   3.69   In the saddle, the trail to East Glacier leads east; a left spur trail climbs the ridge to Scenic Point.

▶5   3.8   Scenic Point; return to trailhead.

East Glacier to Scenic Point

▶1   0.0   Start at the trailhead 0.4 mile down the unpaved road from First Street.

▶2   0.16   Leave the unpaved road and continue west on Mt Henry Trail.

▶3   1.16   Left at trail junction

▶4   2.13   Bald Hill

▶5   6.18   Take the right spur to climb the ridge to Scenic Point.

▶6   6.33   Scenic Point; return to trailhead.

Autumn Creek Trail

Little Dog Mountain, at 8,610 feet, looms above the trail, as seen from the parking area at Marias Pass. The Continental Divide transects the highway here at 5,213 feet elevation. The pass is the lowest route through the Rocky Mountains in the area, and it's one that Great Northern Railway engineer John Stevens and Blackfeet Indian guide Coonsah found ideal for the westward expansion of train tracks in 1889. A statue of Stevens and the Marias Pass Obelisk adorn the parking area.

Best Time

The trail is best skied December through March when snow piles up 6 feet deep. As a summer trail, Autumn Creek is poorly maintained and has several challenging creek crossings in summer—no bridges exist along this trail.

Finding the Trail

On US 2, at the Marias Pass Summit, the trail begins on the northwest side of the highway; a large parking area on the highway's southeast side has pit toilets and historical markers. Use caution when crossing the highway and the railroad tracks. Look for orange and white markers on a tree, and proceed a few feet to find the metal trailhead sign at the forest edge. Leave a shuttle vehicle west of Marias Pass at mile marker 193.8 at a pull-off along the south side of the highway and see the trail's end, a wide, steep jeep trail, on the north side of the highway.

TRAIL USE
Cross-country skiing

LENGTH
5.8 miles, 4–5 hours

VERTICAL FEET
-700'

DIFFICULTY
1 2 3 **4** 5

TRAIL TYPE
Point-to-point

SURFACE TYPE
Snow

START
N48° 19.117'
W113° 21.197'

END
N48° 17.454'
W113° 24.932'

FEATURES
Flora
Secluded
Geologic Interest
Historic Interest
Wildlife

FACILITIES
Pit toilet

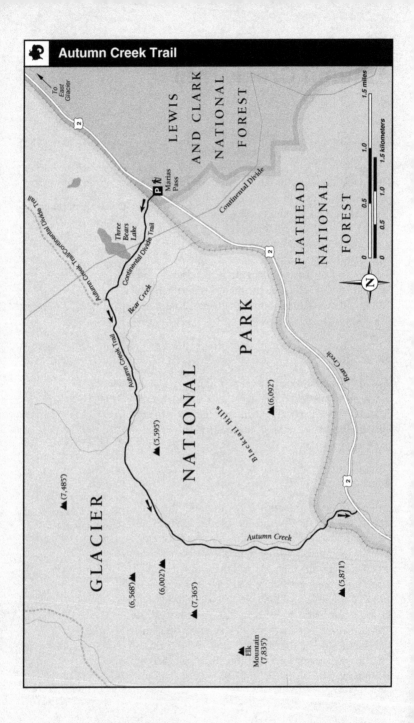

LEWIS AND CLARK NATIONAL FOREST

FLATHEAD NATIONAL FOREST

GLACIER NATIONAL PARK

To East Glacier

Continental Divide Trail

Autumn Creek Trail/Continental Divide Trail

Autumn Creek Trail

Continental Divide Trail

Three Bears Lake

Marias Pass

Continental Divide

Bear Creek

Bear Creek

Blackfoot Hills

Autumn Creek

▲ (7,485')

(6,568') ▲

▲ (6,002')

▲ (7,365')

▲ (5,595')

▲ (6,092)

▲ (5,871')

Elk Mountain (7,835')

1.5 miles
1.0
0.5
0

1.5 kilometers
1.0
0.5
0

N

Trail Description

The ski trail slips through a pine forest to the western edge of the small-acreage Three Bears Lake and the frozen waters of Bear Creek, and along the Continental Divide Trail for just less than a mile. The park service requests that snowshoers "maintain separate tracks for skiing and snowshoeing wherever possible" so the ski tracks are not spoiled—the route is wide enough for snowshoeing next to ski tracks.

At the T, turn left/southwest and keep sight of the orange metal trail markers nailed to trees. The trail glides gently between Little Dog Mountain and the Blacktail Hills, mostly among stocky Douglas fir and lodgepole pine trees. The trail crosses several creek beds, which are frozen or dry in winter—use caution and cross one skier at a time. The overall drop in elevation makes for easy skiing; however, depending on conditions and skiers' abilities, the trail can provide challenges. Many trail users ski or snowshoe into the 3-mile area and return to the trailhead at Marias Pass for a fine day of touring.

The mountain cirque reveals the realm of mountain goats, blue grouse, and black-capped chickadees, winter residents among the trees and lichen-covered rocks in the meadows below Elk

Flathead Avalanche Advisory Information (800-526-5329) details changing snowpack conditions and winter weather forecasts.

Flora

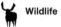
Wildlife

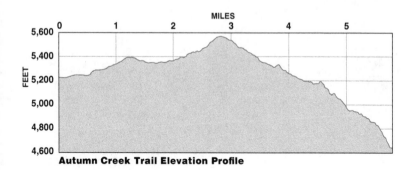
Autumn Creek Trail Elevation Profile

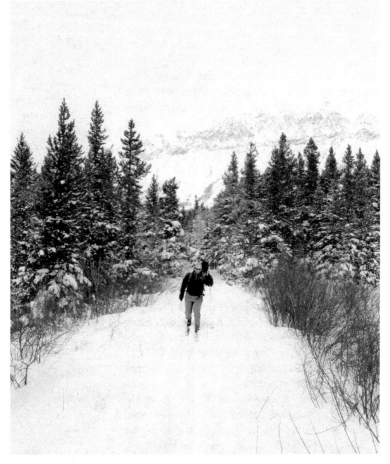

Autumn Creek Trail, *shown here at -10°F, is best skied or snowshoed with a guide from Izaak Walton Inn.*

Marias Pass was named for the Marias River, so named in 1805 by Captain Meriwether Lewis for his cousin and, some speculate, his fiancée, Maria Wood. The Blackfeet called it the Bear River. Autumn Creek was named for its brilliantly colored fall foliage, specifically quaking aspen, shimmering in autumn sunshine.

NOTES

Little Dog Mountain honors Blackfeet Chief Little Dog, or "Imitaikoan" in Blackfeet, once notorious for raiding a covered wagon trail on the Oregon Trail and later known as a promoter of peace, even returning a dozen stolen horses to Fort Benton, a few days' ride east on the Missouri River.

Mountain. Steer clear of avalanche paths streaking off the 7,835-foot Elk Mountain and its eastern neighbor, a 7,485-foot unnamed peak. Incredibly photogenic, this cirque has large "picnic" boulders, perfect for spring ski picnics.

For trail users who are not confident in their route-finding skills, note that experienced guides from Izaak Walton Inn lead trips along Autumn Creek Trail, break trail if necessary, carry emergency radio and gear, and assist with vehicle shuttling. Ski and snowshoe rentals are available at Izaak Walton Inn, which is a 1939 railway inn at Essex, just outside the park boundary near the Walton Ranger Station.

MILESTONES

▶1	0.0	Start from Marias Pass.
▶2	0.75	Ski past Three Bears Lake.
▶3	1.2	At the T, turn left/southwest along Autumn Creek Trail. (Note that the Continental Divide Trail heads right/north.)
▶4	2.8	Highest point on trail; see the mountain cirque; look for the orange ski trail markers nailed to trees.
▶5	3.3	Continue the gentle downhill following the Autumn Creek drainage.
▶6	3.7	Look across and uphill to find the orange trail markers to cross this creek (frozen and mostly dry in winter).
▶7	5.3	Remove skis to cross the railroad tracks; follow the jeep-width trail left/downhill.
▶8	5.8	End at US 2 at mile marker 193.8.

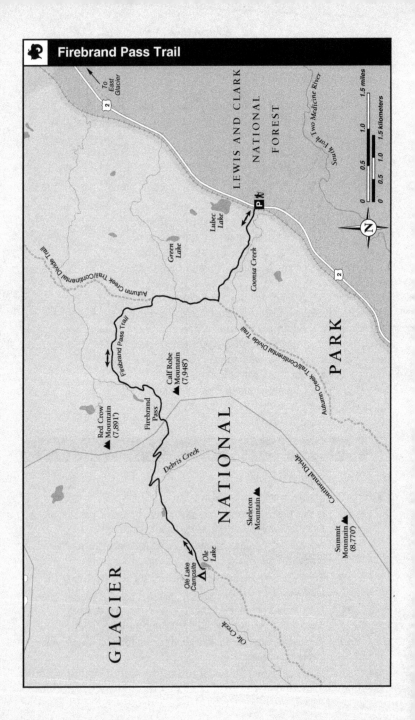

Firebrand Pass Trail

From the 6,951-foot Firebrand Pass, astonishing views east to the plains and north, south, and west into remote mountains both inside and outside the park reward hikers. The hike crosses distinct environments as it climbs from near the Continental Divide and up 2,213 feet to Firebrand Pass.

Best Time

The upper portion of the trail stays blanketed by snow until July. Midsummer through early October, the trail is fully accessible and is a lovely fall hike.

Finding the Trail

From US 2, 4.2 highway miles east of Marias Pass at what's locally known as the False Summit, see mile marker 203 on the southeast side of the road. A gravel parking area on the highway's northwest side is large enough for about 10 vehicles and is between the highway and the railroad tracks. Use extreme caution when crossing the active train tracks. See the corner fence post, wire fencing, trailhead signs, and trail leading west. (Note that Firebrand Pass Food & Ale is at mile marker 206 and is the closest public facility to the trailhead.)

Trail Description

At the trailhead, a marshy area attracts waterfowl, beavers, and moose. Initially, the route follows Coonsa Creek, named for Salish Indian Koonsa, or Red Heart, whose storied past includes 1880s

TRAIL USE
Day hiking

LENGTH
10.26 or 16.0 miles, 4–6 hours

VERTICAL FEET
±2,213'

DIFFICULTY
1 2 3 **4** 5

TRAIL TYPE
Out-and-back

SURFACE TYPE
Dirt, gravel, snow, and ice

START & END
N48° 22.301'
W113° 16.768'0

FEATURES
Flora
Secluded
Geologic Interest
Historic Interest
Wildlife
Birds

FACILITIES
Pit toilets (4.2 miles west of trailhead at Marias Pass)

 Wildlife

Historic Interest

Birds

Flora

Wildlife

Steep

adventures with the law and who was reportedly murdered in 1888. The peak directly ahead is Calf Robe Mountain, with neighbors The Mummy, Summit Mountain, and Little Dog Mountain to the left.

At 0.2 mile, the trail descends slightly into aspens, where black-capped chickadees trill and Cooper's hawks hunt the meadow-forest interface. Spruce grouse might startle hikers when the low flyers panic and zoom across the shady trail. This is grizzly bear country, so be aware, be loud, and be on the lookout for other ursine brethren: black bears, attracted to late-summer feasts, nibble huckleberries, thimbleberries, wild gooseberry, twisted stalk, baneberry, and mountain ash. The Marias pack of gray wolves frequents this area, too, as they hunt rodents, deer, and elk.

At 1.5 miles, the junction with Autumn Creek Trail/Continental Divide Trail sends hikers right/north and following its namesake for a mile out of the forest and into meadows of harebell, wild buckwheat, and noisy Mormon crickets. The next junction, a left/west turn onto Firebrand Pass Trail, begins the climb. Flora changes quickly from subalpine to alpine as elevation increases from 5,500 to 6,951 feet in 2.4 miles. Fortunate flower lovers may see the Montana state flower, the bitterroot

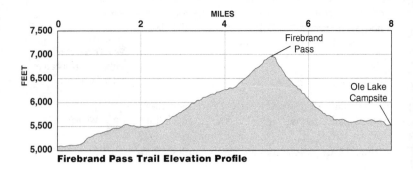

Firebrand Pass Trail Elevation Profile

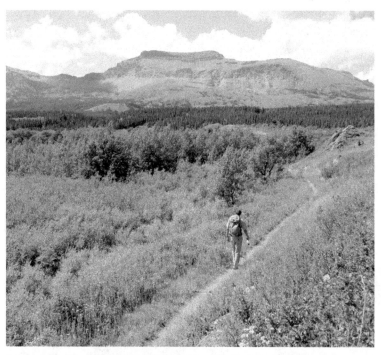

Firebrand Pass *is a brief but challenging trail that offers views into the 200-square-mile Badger–Two Medicine area.*

(*Lewisia rediviva*)—a rare sighting in Glacier. The pink perennial enjoys the gravelly, dry soil here. American Indians collected the root in spring as a food staple, boiled it, and could survive on a small, 2.8-ounce-per-day portion.

 Flora

The trail wraps Calf Robe Mountain's eastern flank. Views become increasingly incredible. To the south is the 115,000-acre Badger–Two Medicine area, sacred to Blackfeet Indians and adjacent to the 1.5-million-acre Bob Marshall Wilderness Complex. Together, Glacier National Park; the designated wilderness complex; and an additional 1 million acres of roadless national forest, private, and Bureau of Land Management land comprise a

 Historic Interest

A firebrand is a flaming piece of wood launched from a wildfire and sent ahead of the fire. Firebrands increase the size of wildland fires by literally leaps and bounds, as happened with the great fires a century ago.

5-million-acre roadless area on the Rocky Mountain Front that is the largest, most intact wild ecosystem in the United States.

Firebrand Pass sits in a breezy saddle between Calf Robe and Red Crow Mountains. The trail continues down a steep decline 3 miles to Ole Lake and Campsite and exits at Fielding–Coal Creek Trailhead for a total of 23.25 miles, mostly in heavy timber. The Firebrand Pass area remains the most spectacular 5 miles.

🚶 MILESTONES

▶1	0.0	Start from the Lubec Trailhead to Autumn Creek Trail and Firebrand Pass Trail.
▶2	1.5	Junction with Autumn Creek Trail; turn right/north on Autumn Creek Trail.
▶3	2.45	Junction with Firebrand Pass Trail; turn left/west.
▶4	5.13	Firebrand Pass. Turn around or continue to Ole Lake.
▶5	8.0	Ole Lake and campground. Return to trailhead.

NOTES

The Lubec Trailhead is named for a former 1913 ranger station about 0.45 mile west of the parking area, beyond the closed dirt road leading west. The Lubec Ranger Station was burned down in 1980 and never rebuilt.

Opposite: *Several small and large waterfalls splash trailside along the Two Medicine Pass Trail to Cobalt Lake.*

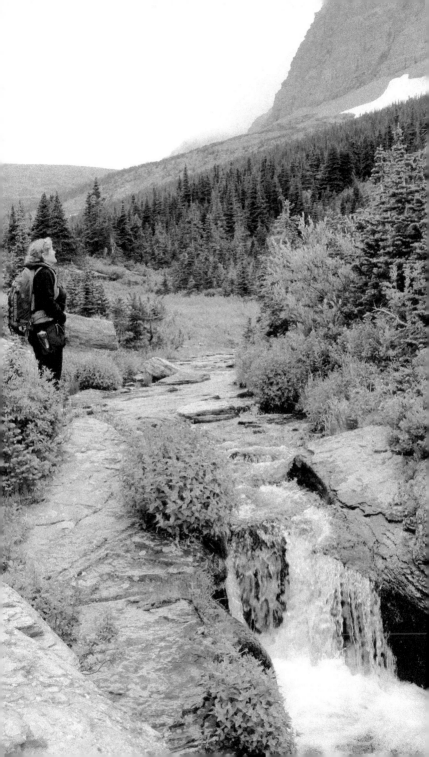

Many Glacier Area

Many Glacier Area

T he Many Glacier area is often visitors' favorite valley of Glacier, thanks in part to the lovely Many Glacier Hotel and its beach, dining room, and ice-cream parlor; the Glacier Park Boat Company's tour boats across Swiftcurrent Lake and Lake Josephine; and the plentiful wildlife that roams here. Visitors often sit on the hotel deck and watch moose or bears— no binoculars needed! At the road's terminus is the Swiftcurrent Motor Inn and Cabins and Many Glacier Campground. Several hikes depart from the motor inn area or the campground and lead into the glorious backcountry, where, by late July, huckleberries begin to ripen under the high-alpine sun. It's from the Many Glacier Valley, too, that visitors often catch their first views of real glaciers, visible from the drive westward into the valley. Drivers must be aware that the road into the valley initially crosses Blackfeet Indian lands, where horse and cattle roam the open range. Drivers must be on high alert for cattle and horses because the ranchlands here on the Blackfeet Reservation are not always fenced, resulting in cattle and horses grazing along the roadways. It is the driver's responsibility to watch out for stock on the 1.5-million-acre Blackfeet Indian Reservation.

The Many Glacier area provides a remarkable glimpse at the geologic crossroads in Glacier. Along the hike to Grinnell Glacier, the trail passes above Grinnell Lake with its vibrant turquoise hue, colored by the glacial till or flour that's scoured from the movement of the glaciers above. Near the base of Grinnell Glacier, visitors stand upon 1,600-million- to 800-million-year-old rock—Precambrian stromatolites, which are blue-green algae fossils that now look like huge rock cabbages yet are evidence of Proterozoic life in the Belt Sea. Towering over the valley is Mount Altyn and its red argillite and blue-green quartzite shoulders, an exemplary display of rock that was compressed under seawater to form Precambrian mudstone. Miners seeking their fortunes dug into the mountainsides looking for copper among the peaks surrounding the Many Glacier Valley, and populated the boomtown of Altyn, on the shore of Cracker Lake, where between 1897 and 1902 nearly 800 people lived.

Opposite and overleaf: *The Many Glacier area's eight trailheads lead to backcountry glaciers, lakes, waterfalls, and even a man-made tunnel through a mountain pass.*

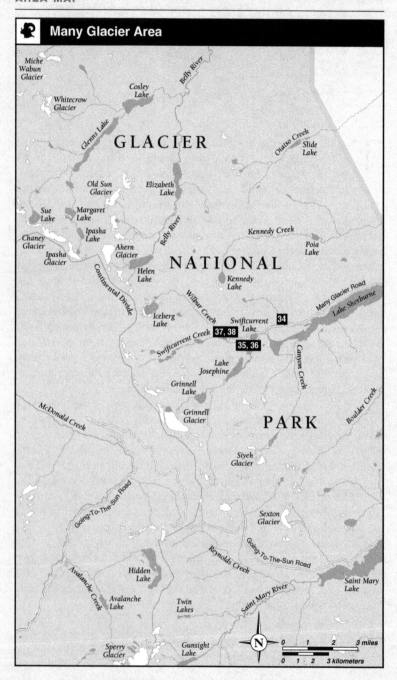

Many Glacier Area

Miche Wabun Glacier

Whitecrow Glacier

Cosley Lake

Belly River

Glenns Lake

GLACIER

Ohatso Creek

Slide Lake

Old Sun Glacier

Elizabeth Lake

Sue Lake

Margaret Lake

Ipasha Lake

Chaney Glacier

Ipasha Glacier

Ahern Glacier

Belly River

Kennedy Creek

Poia Lake

NATIONAL

Helen Lake

Kennedy Lake

Continental Divide

Iceberg Lake

Wilbur Creek

Swiftcurrent Lake

34

Many Glacier Road

Lake Sherburne

37, 38

Swiftcurrent Creek

35, 36

Lake Josephine

Canyon Creek

Grinnell Lake

McDonald Creek

Grinnell Glacier

PARK

Boulder Creek

Siyeh Glacier

Going-To-The-Sun Road

Sexton Glacier

Avalanche Creek

Hidden Lake

Reynolds Creek

Going-To-The-Sun Road

Saint Mary Lake

Avalanche Lake

Twin Lakes

Saint Mary River

N

Sperry Glacier

Gunsight Lake

0 1 2 3 miles

0 1 2 3 kilometers

TRAIL FEATURES TABLE

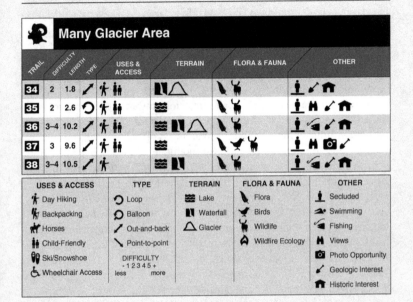

Many Glacier Area

TRAIL	DIFFICULTY	LENGTH	TYPE	USES & ACCESS	TERRAIN	FLORA & FAUNA	OTHER
34	2	1.8	Out-and-back	Day Hiking, Child-Friendly	Waterfall, Glacier	Flora, Wildlife	Secluded, Geologic Interest, Historic Interest
35	2	2.6	Loop	Day Hiking, Child-Friendly	Lake	Flora, Wildlife	Secluded, Views, Fishing, Historic Interest
36	3–4	10.2	Out-and-back	Day Hiking, Child-Friendly	Lake, Waterfall, Glacier	Flora, Wildlife	Secluded, Fishing, Geologic Interest, Historic Interest
37	3	9.6	Out-and-back	Day Hiking, Child-Friendly	Lake	Flora, Birds, Wildlife	Secluded, Views, Photo Opportunity, Geologic Interest
38	3–4	10.5	Out-and-back	Day Hiking	Lake, Waterfall	Flora, Wildlife	Secluded, Fishing, Geologic Interest, Historic Interest

USES & ACCESS	TYPE	TERRAIN	FLORA & FAUNA	OTHER
Day Hiking	Loop	Lake	Flora	Secluded
Backpacking	Balloon	Waterfall	Birds	Swimming
Horses	Out-and-back	Glacier	Wildlife	Fishing
Child-Friendly	Point-to-point		Wildfire Ecology	Views
Ski/Snowshoe	DIFFICULTY			Photo Opportunity
Wheelchair Access	- 1 2 3 4 5 +			Geologic Interest
	less more			Historic Interest

Permits and Maps

No permit is required to hike inside Glacier; however, a Blackfeet Conservation/Recreation Use Permit is required for hiking, biking, horseback riding, and fishing on the reservation (call 406-338-7207 for more information). A fishing permit is not required to fish in Glacier, but a Montana fishing license is required outside the park and is for sale at most outfitters, sporting goods stores, and some grocery stores. Fishing is catch-and-release only in certain areas for cutthroat trout—check with the entrance stations or ranger stations for details. The daily catch-and-possession limit is five fish, with a maximum of two cutthroat trout, two burbot (ling), one northern pike, two mountain whitefish, five lake whitefish, five kokanee salmon, five grayling, five rainbow trout, and five lake trout. The following creeks are closed to fishing for their entire length: Ole, Park, Muir, Coal, Nyack, Fish, Lee, Otatso, Boulder, and Kennedy Creeks.

Free park maps are available at entrance stations. Each of the park's lodging properties offers rudimentary local-area maps with details of trailhead access. Excellent maps are available for purchase at the in-park bookstores, gift shops, and grocery stores, as well as through the Glacier National Park Conservancy's bookstore in the West Glacier train depot, sporting goods shops, and general stores outside the park and online.

Opposite: *The Grinnell Glacier Trail along Lake Josephine climbs to three remaining glaciers, including Grinnell, Salamander, and Gem.*

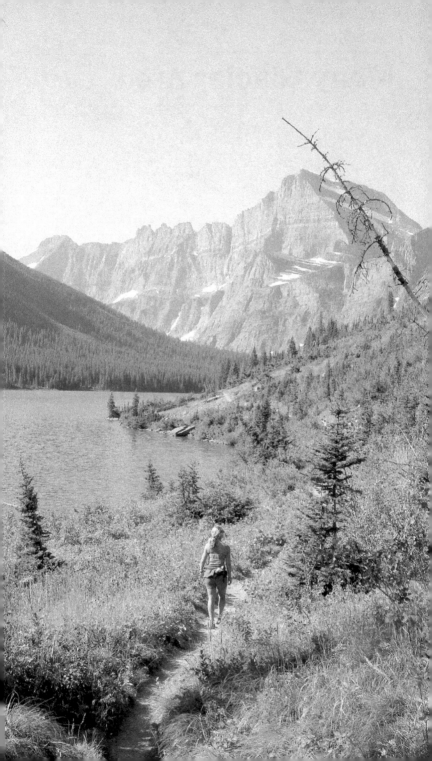

Many Glacier Area

TRAIL 37

Day hiking, youth-
friendly
9.6 miles
Out-and-back
Difficulty 1 2 **3** 4 5

This hike, mostly along moderate terrain, leads westward where the jagged horizon of the glacial arête above is called the Ptarmigan Wall and where below lies well-loved Iceberg Lake. It's often still iced over through June but is one of the park's foremost attractions—for humans and bears! While this trail is susceptible to closure due to bear activity, it remains one of the park's most memorable traces.

TRAIL 38

Day hiking
10.5 miles
Out-and-back
Difficulty 1 2 **3** 4 5

This 1930s man-made tunnel is quite a backcountry engineering feat, created so horses and hikers could move from one valley to the next without traversing a dangerous pass. The huckleberry-laden hike to the tunnel unveils wildflower-thick meadows, waterfalls, turquoise lakes, and jagged mountains; it's well worth every foot of the 5.8-mile climb.

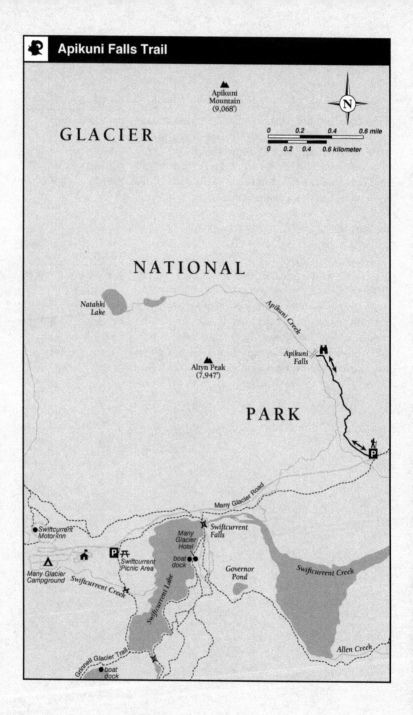

Apikuni
Mountain
(9,068')

GLACIER

0   0.2   0.4   0.6 mile
0   0.2   0.4   0.6 kilometer

NATIONAL

Natahki
Lake

Apikuni Creek

Apikuni
Falls

Altyn Peak
(7,947')

PARK

Many Glacier Road

Swiftcurrent
Motor Inn

Many
Glacier
Hotel

Swiftcurrent
Falls

Swiftcurrent
Picnic Area

boat
dock

Governor
Pond

Swiftcurrent Creek

Many Glacier
Campground

Swiftcurrent Creek

Swiftcurrent Lake

Allen Creek

Grinnell Glacier Trail

boat
dock

Apikuni Falls Trail (aka Appekunny Falls Trail)

Fantastic views of Salamander Glacier and Grinnell Glacier loom above and across Many Glacier Valley and are visible from several viewpoints along the hike up to Apikuni Falls. Gem Glacier also comes into view as hikers look over their left/west shoulders to the Garden Wall's collection of receding glaciers. Glaciers formed this valley, with its 4,750-foot elevation changes, from the valley floor at 4,800 feet elevation to the high point, Mount Gould's summit at 9,553 feet elevation. This hike, however, climbs only 650 feet, from a valley to the base of Apikuni Falls on the east skirt of 7,947-foot Altyn Peak. The 9,068-foot Apikuni Mountain hovers behind the falls. Both peaks are visible from the trailhead, although the falls remain hidden until 0.8 mile. There is an easy scramble from trail's end to the falls, 100 steps farther.

Best Time

The trail becomes snow-free in late May in most years. Once summer temperatures heat up the park, this trail is best hiked in the morning, since it climbs a south-facing slope. Trees provide some shade while you climb a fairly steep grade to the falls.

Finding the Trail

The trailhead is on the north side of Many Glacier Road at mile marker 10.4, just 2.4 miles west of the park entrance station. It is well marked with the sign for Poia Lake Trailhead/Apikuni Falls Trailhead (also known as Appekunny Falls). The parking area is large enough for a dozen vehicles.

TRAIL USE
Day hiking, child-friendly

LENGTH
1.8 miles, 1–2 hours

VERTICAL FEET
±650'

DIFFICULTY
1 **2** 3 4 5

TRAIL TYPE
Out-and-back

SURFACE TYPE
Dirt and gravel

START & END
N48° 48.326'
W113° 38.072'

FEATURES
Flora
Secluded
Geologic Interest
Historic Interest
Wildlife
Waterfall
Glaciers

FACILITIES
Ranger station
Lodging
Restaurants
Stores
Interpretive center
Campgrounds

235

Glacier National Park's geological formations are revealed here. Precambrian Age Belt Series sedimentary rock from the shallow Belt Sea dates from some 1,600 million to 800 million years ago.

Historic Interest

Waterfall

Trail Description

The trail initially leads northwest across a wildflower-strewn meadow—deceptively gentle terrain, for soon the trail climbs unceasingly to the falls. As you take a breather from the climb, notice the valley immediately below and south across Many Glacier Road. This is the site of the once-thriving mining town, Altyn, on the shore of Cracker Lake. Between 1897 and 1902, nearly 800 people lived here, seeking fortunes in copper mining. Most of the boomtown remains are underwater; the Lake Sherburne Dam forced Swiftcurrent Creek into a reservoir, flooding the town in 1921. Now the Bureau of Reclamation manages the irrigation and recreation water as it flows to the Milk River.

Indeed, water gushing over Apikuni Falls is snowmelt from Altyn Peak and Apikuni Mountain, water that drains into Natahki Lake, then Apikuni Creek and over the falls and eventually into Lake Sherburne. As the trail switchbacks upward, you will see where spur routes depart to overlooks—keep children away from these cliffs, and note that the footing can be precarious near the cliffs. It's best to stay on the main trail, as you have many viewpoints available throughout the hike. You

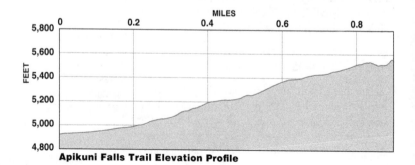

Apikuni Falls Trail Elevation Profile

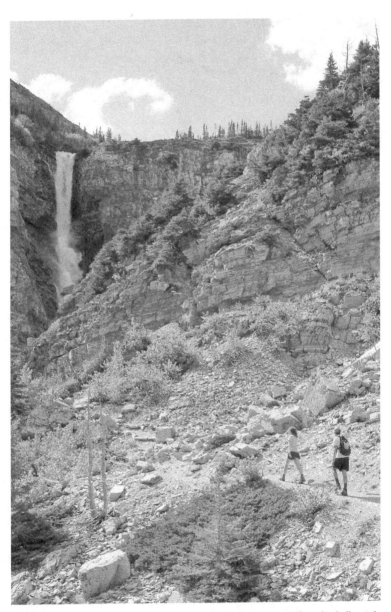

Apikuni Falls *tumbles among Precambrian Belt Series sedimentary rock from the shallow Belt Sea, dating 1,600 to 800 million years old.*

NOTES

Apikuni, the Blackfeet word for Far Off White Robe, Spotted Robe, or Far-Away Robe (depending upon the translation), is the name the Blackfeet gave to explorer and historian James Willard Schultz, who wrote about the region for *Field & Stream* magazine. Apikuni is sometimes spelled Appekunny.

Wildlife

might see both mountain goats and bighorn sheep on the shoulder of Altyn Peak. Bears frequent the area as well.

Wildflowers bloom, from the sunny meadow's sticky geranium to aspen-shaded beargrass, Indian paintbrush, and strawberry—and then pine-shaded wild rose, columbine, huckleberry, and clematis.

Wildflowers

The dirt trail, littered with blue and pink rock, can become slick if wet. The rock, red argillite and blue-green quartzite, became compressed under seawater

Geologic Interest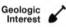

to form Precambrian mudstone. Look to Mount Altyn for a brilliant display of the red argillite, especially during early morning and evening lighting.

🚶 MILESTONES

▶1 0.0   Start from Many Glacier Road 2.4 miles west of the entrance station.

▶2 0.1   Cross Apikuni Flats and begin climbing.

▶3 0.2   Spur trail to Apikuni Creek

▶4 0.25 Overlook

▶5 0.8   Trees become sparse—see and hear the falls just ahead.

▶6 0.9   Apikuni Falls. Return to trailhead.

Swiftcurrent Lake Nature Trail

Incredible views with every blink reward hikers on this route circumnavigating the aquamarine Swiftcurrent Lake. Aspen groves give way to evergreens, riparian areas, and a pebbled beach. While the Swiftcurrent Lake Nature Trail is a pleasant 2.6-mile loop, it is easy to add an additional 0.8 mile with a spur trail to Lake Josephine and significantly different views. The trails are well marked; however, pay close attention to each junction. National Park Service pamphlets are available at the trailhead for a small donation and provide useful and interesting details of the Many Glacier Valley.

Best Time

The trail opens with road access into Many Glacier Valley, usually May through October, although in early spring, snow and mud cover portions of the trail. Pay attention to trail closures or postings for grizzly bear activity.

Finding the Trail

From Many Glacier Road/Glacier Route 3, 0.4 mile west of the Many Glacier Hotel turnoff, the trailhead begins in Many Glacier Picnic Area on the south side of the road. Park here.

Trail Description

Swiftcurrent Lake Trail begins on Grinnell Glacier Trail, on the southernmost point of the horseshoe-shaped picnic loop at a wide graveled area. Many

TRAIL USE
Day hiking,
youth-friendly

LENGTH
2.6 miles, 2–3 hours

VERTICAL FEET
±24'

DIFFICULTY
1 **2** 3 4 5

TRAIL TYPE
Loop

SURFACE TYPE
Dirt and gravel

START & END
N48° 47.827'
W113° 40.106'

FEATURES
Lakes
Flora
Secluded
Geologic Interest
Historic Interest
Wildlife
Views

FACILITIES
Ranger station
Lodging, Restaurants
Stores, Gas
Interpretive center
Picnic area
Campgrounds, Showers
Boat dock, Tour boat
Rental canoes

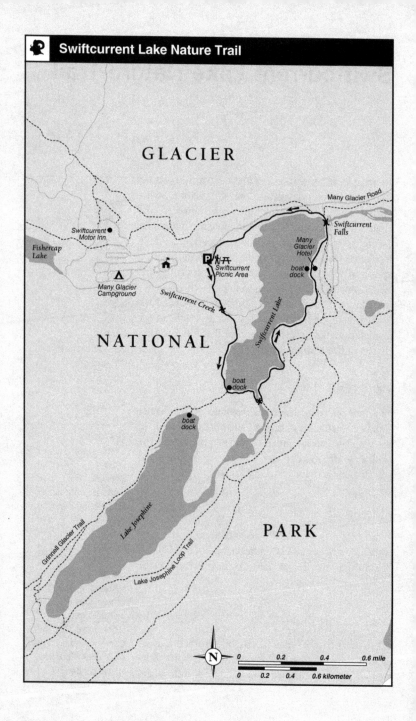

Swiftcurrent Lake Nature Trail

GLACIER

Many Glacier Road

Swiftcurrent
Motor Inn

Fishercap
Lake

Swiftcurrent
Falls

Many
Glacier
Hotel

boat
dock

Many Glacier
Campground

Swiftcurrent
Picnic Area

Swiftcurrent Creek

NATIONAL

Swiftcurrent Lake

boat
dock

boat
dock

Lake Josephine

Grinnell Glacier Trail

PARK

Lake Josephine Loop Trail

N

| 0 | 0.2 | 0.4 | 0.6 mile |

| 0 | 0.2 | 0.4 | 0.6 kilometer |

Glacier Hotel guests can enter the loop trail from the hotel beach. This description is for a counterclockwise loop hike. As you cross the Swiftcurrent Creek footbridge, look upstream for views of Mount Wilbur and Bishops Cap along the Continental Divide. The trail leads south into the forest of lodgepole pine and subalpine fir. A look to the east across the lake provides exquisite views of Many Glacier Hotel. You might see the horse concession cowboys on the hill behind the hotel heading out on trail rides to Cracker Lake, another lovely Glacier route but best via horseback because of the high traffic of outfitters' steeds. You can see 9,376-foot Allen Mountain to the south and 8,404-foot Mount Wynn directly east.

The trail paralleling Swiftcurrent Lake's west shore is relatively flat. You might see moose in or near the shallow water of the 1- by 0.5-mile lake, as bull or cow and calf submerge for underwater sedges. Snowberry, serviceberry, thimbleberry, and huckleberry bushes fill the understory, along with lavender aster and queen-cup flowers.

As you round the southern end of the lake, the view changes from lake and hotel backdropped by Altyn Peak to lake and several mountains, all part of the Lewis Range. The pyramid-shaped Grinnell Point is closest to the lake's west shore. Behind Grinnell Point are (left to right) 9,553-foot Mount

The Blackfeet called this area Waterfalls, or *Ohpskunakaxi*. The Blackfeet term for "lots of ice," or many glaciers, is *akokokutoi*.

 Views

 Wildlife

 Flora

Lake

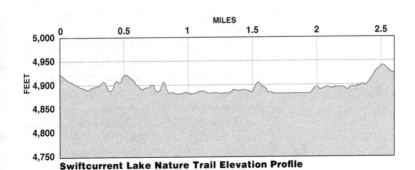
Swiftcurrent Lake Nature Trail Elevation Profile

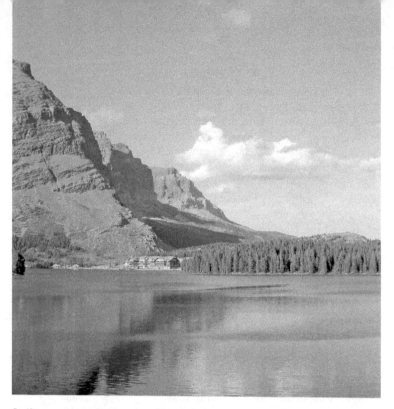

Swiftcurrent Lake Trail *gently wends around the lake, providing picture-worthy vistas, including Many Glacier Hotel, which was opened in 1915 by the Great Northern Railway.*

Gould, 9,321-foot Mount Wilbur, the Garden Wall, and 8,770-foot Mount Henkel.

The trail leads north past a few employee cabins and the boathouse for *Chief Two Guns* tour boat before reaching the Many Glacier Hotel beach and boat dock.

The final stretch of the loop includes a must-stop for ice cream, Heidi's Snack Shop and Espresso Stand, in the basement of Many Glacier Hotel, before tackling the pebble beach walk and momentarily the shoulder of the street as you cross over Swiftcurrent Falls. The trail again hugs the shoreline heading west and parallels Many Glacier Road to return to the trailhead. Look north to Altyn Peak's shoulder—bears and bighorn sheep often graze here.

Wildlife

MILESTONES

▶1   0.0   Start from the picnic and day parking area along Many Glacier Road/Glacier Route 3.

▶2   0.24   Footbridge over Swiftcurrent Creek

▶3   0.7   Boat dock and Lake Josephine spur trail

▶4   0.85   Footbridge then junction with Lake Josephine Loop Trail; stay left, heading north.

▶5   1.7   Boat dock and beach in front of Many Glacier Hotel

▶6   1.92   Bridge over Swiftcurrent Falls

▶7   2.6   Trailhead, parking, and picnic area

NOTES

The chalet-style Many Glacier Hotel, built by the Great Northern Railway on the eastern shore of Swiftcurrent Lake, opened July 2, 1915. The hotel currently opens June–September each year.

Moose munch underwater vegetation and willows, seemingly oblivious to humans; however, they are unpredictable, dangerous mammals best observed from a distance or from the deck of Many Glacier Hotel.

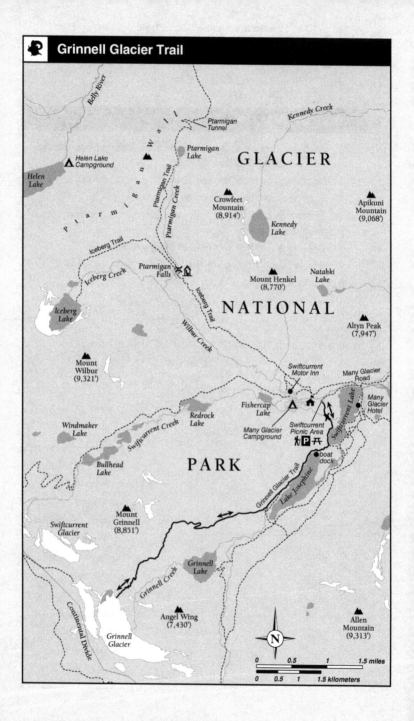

Grinnell Glacier Trail

As one of the most picturesque and popular hikes in the park, the trail to Grinnell Glacier exhibits crystalline lakes, jagged peaks, and, at trail's terminus, three of the park's famed glaciers: Grinnell, Salamander, and Gem. At trailside are luscious huckleberries, fragrant wildflowers, and a trail seemingly paved in pink argillite. Ancient rock chips of metamorphosed mudstone from the Belt Formation glisten deep red when wet. Best of all are this hike's options: Either hike the entire 5.1 miles to Upper Grinnell Lake, or ride the tour boats to shorten the one-way trip by 1.7 miles. For details on the tour boat option, see the sidebar on page 247.

Best Time

The trail climbs from the valley floor and into the snowy realms of the park, with the upper section opening July through September, when dazzling wildflowers outline the vibrant turquoise lakes. The trail's middle and upper regions tend to get hot by midsummer, so it's best to begin the hike in the morning. Check tour boat hours if taking the cruises.

Finding the Trail

From Many Glacier Road/Glacier Route 3, at 0.4 mile west of the Many Glacier Hotel turnoff, the trailhead begins in the Many Glacier Picnic Area, on the south side of the road. Park here. Grinnell Glacier Trail (also the Swiftcurrent Lake Trail) begins on the southernmost point of the horseshoe-shaped picnic loop at a wide graveled area.

TRAIL USE
Day hiking, child-friendly
LENGTH
10.2 miles, 5–7 hours
VERTICAL FEET
±1,600'
DIFFICULTY
1 2 **3 4** 5
TRAIL TYPE
Out-and-back
SURFACE TYPE
Dirt and gravel
START & END
N48° 47.827'
W113° 40.106'
BOAT DOCK:
N48° 47.958'
W113° 39.819'

FEATURES
Flora, Secluded
Geologic Interest
Historic Interest
Wildlife, Lakes, Fishing
Waterfall, Glacier

FACILITIES
Ranger station
Lodging, Restaurants
Stores, Gas
Interpretive center
Picnic area
Campgrounds, Showers
Boat dock, Tour boat
Rental canoes

Trail Description

Lake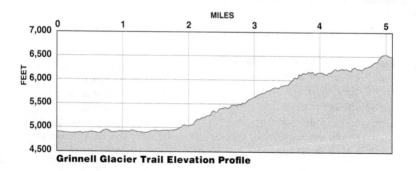

Wildlife

Historic Interest

Lake

Wildlife

The initial 0.7-mile trek cruises along the west shore of Swiftcurrent Lake (see Swiftcurrent Lake Trail, Trail 35), a lovely and gentle walk where moose and bear reside—hike in groups, make plenty of noise, carry bear spray, and know how to use it. At the south end of the lake, you'll find the boat dock and a 400-yard walk to Lake Josephine over the hill that separates the bejeweled lakes. It's possible that Lake Josephine was named for a miner's mule, Josephine. The lake also may have been named for homesteader Josephine Doody.

Near the head of Lake Josephine, the trail ascends quickly. A reward awaits: Grinnell Lake sparkles far below. An optional 0.75-mile hike from Lake Josephine's southern boat dock explores Grinnell Lake, where a twice-daily naturalist-led walk is available via the tour boat operation. Its vibrant turquoise hue is due to the glacial till or flour that's scoured from the movement of the glaciers above. As you hike, listen for the sound of bighorn sheep, as the rams' skull-crashing sparring occurs during the fall competition for ewes. It sounds like coconuts clunking together and can be heard a mile away. Bighorns have a thick, bony skull that prevents brain damage despite the power involved in the head-butting collisions.

Grinnell Glacier Trail Elevation Profile

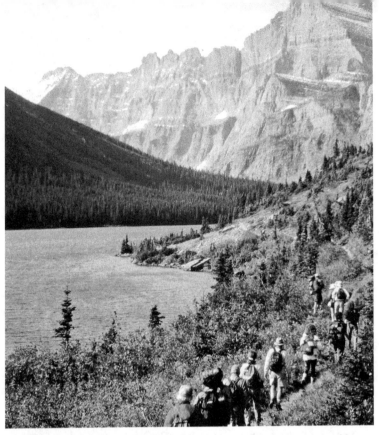

The Grinnell Glacier Trail is studded with turquoise lakes, three glaciers, and plentiful wildlife, including bighorn sheep.

OPTIONS

A fantastic option is to start from the boat dock at Many Glacier Hotel, ride Glacier Park Boats across Swiftcurrent Lake and Lake Josephine, and then hike to the glaciers, eliminating 1.7 miles each way. Total mileage for this option is 8.4, and the trip takes 3–4 hours.

If you choose to ride *Chief Two Guns* from Many Glacier Hotel's boat dock, your hike begins on the wide path between the lakes with an 80-foot climb for 0.2 mile. Boat passengers next board the *Morning Eagle* for an interpretive cruise to the head of Lake Josephine. The boat captain shares local lore about the mines in the area, including the mine shaft above the lake.

Lake	Upper Grinnell Lake and three glaciers are just a brief climb where the trail wends through rock
Glacier	next to Grinnell Falls. As breezes caress the glacial

Lake

Glacier

Waterfall

Geologic Interest

Upper Grinnell Lake and three glaciers are just a brief climb where the trail wends through rock next to Grinnell Falls. As breezes caress the glacial ice, the air cools—pack a jacket. Not only do hikers have intimate views of three glaciers, the Garden Wall, and 9,553-foot Mount Gould, but also at your feet are 1,600-million- to 800-million-year-old rock—Precambrian stromatolites, blue-green algae fossils that look like huge rock cabbage and are evidence of Proterozoic life in the Belt Sea.

The park forbids climbing on the glacial ice and warns that the lake ice may have hidden fissures where a hiker could fall through.

🚶 MILESTONES

►1	0.0	Start from picnic and day parking area on Many Glacier Road/ Glacier Route 3.
►2	0.24	Footbridge over Swiftcurrent Creek
►3	0.7	Swiftcurrent Upper Boat Dock and Lake Josephine spur trail
►4	0.85	Lake Josephine Boat Dock; hike the lake-hugging trail along the north shore of Lake Josephine.
►5	4.68	Picnic table and pit toilet
►6	5.1	Grinnell Glacier and Upper Grinnell Lake. Return to trailhead.

NOTES

Researchers note that the melt rate of the park's glaciers indicates that no glaciers will exist by the year 2020, and currently fewer than two dozen glaciers larger than 25 acres remain in the park. In 1850, 150 glaciers existed. Once ice recedes to less than 25 acres, it is no longer considered a glacier.

Iceberg Lake

While the first 0.2 mile climbs, sometimes like stairsteps, up 275 feet, don't be intimidated. The rest of the trail is a gentle incline to a glaciated cirque where the ice cloaks the lake well into July. When the aquamarine lake melts, large and small blocks of ice float the 0.5- by 0.3-mile tarn. Note that some maps call this the Ptarmigan Trail or the Iceberg Lake–Ptarmigan Tunnel Trail.

Best Time

Early June–October, this trail is best started in the morning since afternoon sun heats up the trail, much of which is at the treeline; thus, the trail rolls in and out of shade. The intense sun also melts snow—up to a foot per day—so the first 3 miles of Iceberg Lake Trail is one of the earlier high-elevation routes to become snow-free. The final ascent and descent to the lake itself are often snow-covered into July. Because of bear activity, it's best to hike in groups of three or more, make plenty of noise, and complete the hike long before sunset.

Finding the Trail

From the Swiftcurrent Motor Inn, a large TRAIL-HEADS sign is just west of the café. A right/north turn, as the sign indicates, leads into the rental cabin area on a paved road; it's 0.1 mile to the parking and trailhead signs for Iceberg Lake and Ptarmigan Tunnel.

Another trailhead begins near the Many Glacier Hotel, nearly adjacent to the hotel's driveway, on the

TRAIL USE
Day hiking, youth-friendly

LENGTH
9.6 miles, 4–6 hours

VERTICAL FEET
+1,245'/-1,245'

DIFFICULTY
1 2 **3** 4 5

TRAIL TYPE
Out-and-back

SURFACE TYPE
Dirt

START & END
N48° 47.976'
W113° 40.755'

FEATURES
Lake
Birds
Flora
Secluded
Wildlife
Geologic Interest
Views
Photo opportunity

FACILITIES
Campground
Restrooms
Restaurant
Gift/gear shop
Hotel
Ranger station

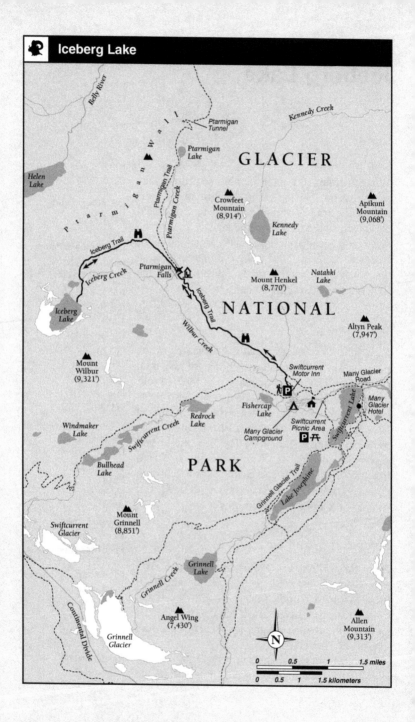

Belly River

Kennedy Creek

Ptarmigan
Tunnel

Ptarmigan
Lake

GLACIER

Helen
Lake

P t a r m i g a n   W a l l

Crowfeet
Mountain
(8,914')

Apikuni
Mountain
(9,068')

Iceberg Trail

Ptarmigan Trail

Ptarmigan Creek

Kennedy
Lake

Iceberg Creek

Ptarmigan
Falls

Natahki
Lake

Iceberg
Lake

Iceberg Trail

Mount Henkel
(8,770')

NATIONAL

Wilbur Creek

Altyn Peak
(7,947')

Mount
Wilbur
(9,321')

Swiftcurrent
Motor Inn

Many Glacier
Road

P

Many
Glacier
Lake

Fishercap
Lake

Swiftcurrent
Picnic Area

Many Glacier
Hotel

Windmaker
Lake

Swiftcurrent Creek

Redrock
Lake

Many Glacier
Campground

P

Swiftcurrent Lake

Bullhead
Lake

PARK

Swiftcurrent
Glacier

Mount
Grinnell
(8,851')

Grinnell Glacier Trail

Lake Josephine

Grinnell
Lake

Grinnell Creek

Continental Divide

Angel Wing
(7,430')

Allen
Mountain
(9,313')

Grinnell
Glacier

N

0   0.5   1   1.5 miles

0   0.5   1   1.5 kilometers

north side of Many Glacier Road and 400 feet west of the turn-in for the hotel. This trailhead adds 1.3 miles to the hike but is often closed due to bear activity.

Trail Description

As you hike, notice on the western horizon a jagged glacial arête called the Ptarmigan Wall (a ptarmigan is a northern grouse, indigenous to the region). Massive glaciers ground away at both sides of these mountains, creating a thin rim along the Continental Divide. One spot actually has been worn by wind and weather such that a hole through the rock is visible, best seen at sunset from the deck of Many Glacier Hotel. Iceberg Lake Trail is surrounded by photogenic peaks. The trail begins on the southern skirt of Altyn Peak, cruises between Mount Wilbur to the south and Mount Henkel then Crowfeet Mountain to the north, and finally curves south to the lake below the Ptarmigan Wall and Iceberg Peak, all part of the Lewis Range of the Northern Rockies.

Grizzly bears frequent the trail. Visitors are welcome to join the daily summer ranger-led hike for both the interpretive information and for the hiking group. The ranger may point out wildlife, such as mountain goats, bighorn sheep, and grizzly bears

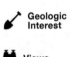

Geologic Interest

Views

Iceberg Lake was called *Kokutoi Omahxikimi,* or "ice lake," by the Blackfeet Indians. Its current and aptly descriptive name probably came from George Bird Grinnell in 1890.

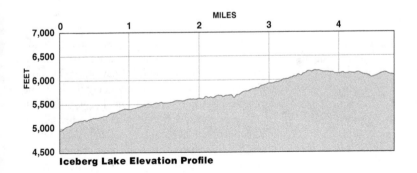

Iceberg Lake Elevation Profile

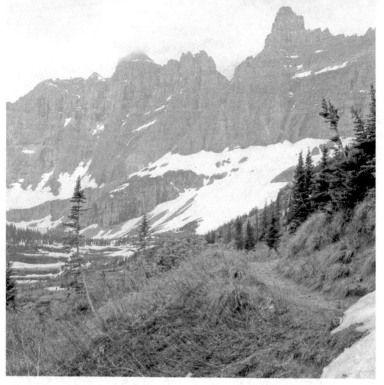

Iceberg Lake Trail, *one of Glacier's most popular backcountry strolls, ambles below the Continental Divide, where icebergs float in the lake even in August and September.*

Wildlife that dig up and eat glacier lily bulbs. As you hike, you may see places where the soil is disturbed or logs are rolled over where bears have sought grubs. Bears also seek the huckleberries, serviceberries, snowberries, thimbleberries, and buffalo berries that thrive in this lodgepole pine and aspen forest and in the wildflower meadows. Brilliant red Indian paintbrush captures your attention, as does the lantern-bright white beargrass waving in the **Flora** breeze. A beargrass bulb blooms about every five to seven years, so some years will have more blossom stalks than others. Interestingly enough, the name "beargrass" is a misnomer; it's neither popular with bears nor a grass. Beargrass is from the lily family; has a large bunch of basal leaves, which do look like grass; and has many tiny flowers at the top of the stalk, which form the puffy bulb of flowers. While

Lewis and Clark got many things right, the naming of beargrass was not one of them. On June 15, 1805, while in today's Bitterroot Mountains of Montana, Lewis wrote, "There is a great abundance of a species of bear-grass which grows on every part of these mountains." Many suggest that beargrass should become the official flower of Glacier.

As the trail rises above most of the trees, look above you to see the mountain goats scampering along the cliffs or lounging in the midday heat. You might see mountain bluebirds flitting between the scrubby trees and hear ground squirrels sounding the alarm that hikers are near. The lake and a small pond below the lake finally come into view. A quick descent to Iceberg Lake cruises through a high alpine meadow that shows evidence of last winter's avalanches.

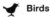 **Birds**

 Lake

🚶 MILESTONES

▶1   0.0   Start at the Swiftcurrent Motor Inn parking area for cabins and trailhead.

▶2   0.24   The trail meets the spur trail from Many Glacier Hotel; turn left/west.

▶3   1.0   Natural benches of red rock provide an amphitheater. Look closely to see wavy designs in the red and green argillite, from ancient waves in a Precambrian-age sea.

▶4   2.0   Look west to see Swiftcurrent Glacier.

▶5   2.38   A trail on the right leads to the outhouse a few steps off the main trail.

▶6   2.58   Ptarmigan Falls and footbridge

▶7   2.66   Junction with Ptarmigan Trail and the route to Ptarmigan Tunnel; stay left for Iceberg Lake.

▶8   3.2   View the cirque surrounding Iceberg Lake and the lower, unnamed icy pond. The trail descends to the pond and Iceberg Creek outlet.

▶9   4.45   Cross Iceberg Creek.

▶10 4.8   Iceberg Lake; return to trailhead.

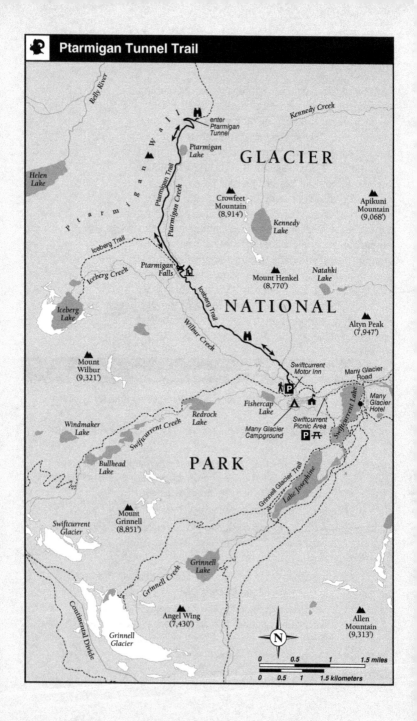

Belly River

Kennedy Creek

enter
Ptarmigan
Tunnel

Ptarmigan Wall

Ptarmigan
Lake

GLACIER

Helen
Lake

Crowfeet
Mountain
(8,914')

Kennedy
Lake

Apikuni
Mountain
(9,068')

Ptarmigan Trail

Ptarmigan Creek

Iceberg Trail

Iceberg Creek

Ptarmigan
Falls

Mount Henkel
(8,770')

Natahki
Lake

NATIONAL

Iceberg
Lake

Iceberg Trail

Wilbur Creek

Altyn Peak
(7,947')

Mount
Wilbur
(9,321')

Swiftcurrent
Motor Inn

Many Glacier
Road

Many Glacier Lake

Fishercap
Lake

Many Glacier Hotel

Windmaker
Lake

Swiftcurrent Creek

Redrock
Lake

Many Glacier
Campground

Swiftcurrent
Picnic Area

Swiftcurrent Lake

PARK

Bullhead
Lake

Grinnell Glacier Trail

Lake Josephine

Swiftcurrent
Glacier

Mount
Grinnell
(8,851')

Grinnell
Lake

Grinnell Creek

Continental Divide

Grinnell
Glacier

Angel Wing
(7,430')

Allen
Mountain
(9,313')

N

| 0 | 0.5 | 1 | 1.5 miles |

| 0 | 0.5 | 1 | 1.5 kilometers |

Ptarmigan Tunnel Trail

A man-made tunnel drilled through a mountain pass in the backcountry is the final destination, yet the hike to Ptarmigan Tunnel is rife with wild-flower-thick meadows, waterfalls, turquoise lakes, and jagged mountains. In early summer, the trail is more difficult, thanks to snow cover, which melts by late July.

Best Time

The trail is passable by mid-July and through October; however, the tunnel isn't opened until snow clears from the trail and tunnel doors, usually late July through late September. Check with the ranger station prior to hiking regarding snow, tunnel doors, and wildlife. The trail is frequently closed due to bear activity.

Finding the Trail

From the Swiftcurrent Motor Inn, look for the large TRAILHEADS sign just west of the café. A right/north turn, as the sign indicates, leads into the rental cabin area on a paved road; it's 0.1 mile to the parking and trailhead signs, which indicate ICEBERG LAKE AND PTARMIGAN TUNNEL.

Another trailhead begins near the Many Glacier Hotel, nearly adjacent to the hotel's driveway, on the north side of Many Glacier Road and 400 feet west of the turn-in for the hotel. This trailhead adds 1.3 miles to the hike but is often closed due to bear activity.

TRAIL USE
Day hiking

LENGTH
10.5 miles, 6–8 hours

VERTICAL FEET
±2,372

DIFFICULTY
1 2 **3 4** 5

TRAIL TYPE
Out-and-back

SURFACE TYPE
Dirt, rock, gravel, and snow

START & END
N48° 47.976'
W113° 40.755'

FEATURES
Flora
Secluded
Geologic Interest
Historic Interest
Wildlife
Lakes
Fishing
Waterfalls

FACILITIES
Ranger station
Lodging
Restaurants
Stores
Interpretive center
Campgrounds
Ranger-led hikes

Trail Description

After the initial 0.35-mile climb from the trailhead, the route cruises for 2 miles through patches of timber and open meadows above the Wilbur Creek Valley to the junction with Ptarmigan Tunnel Trail, a right/north turn. Here's where a steady climb begins. A nearly 2-mile hill climb among huckleberry bushes, beargrass, aspen, lodgepole pine, and subalpine fir rewards hikers with an aquamarine lake back-dropped by a mountain cirque.

Flora

Lake

Fishing at Ptarmigan Lake proves successful—a park permit is not required—although be bear-aware because grizzlies roam here. Bighorn sheep, mountain goats, black bears, marmots, and chipmunks populate the trailside too. From the lakeshore trail, you can often see bighorns and mountain goats climbing on the rocky ledges above the lake. You might see the rock wall at the tunnel as your eyes follow the final 0.9-mile, 735-foot climb along three switchbacks. The rock outside the tunnel is a different shade.

Wildlife

Once at the tunnel, take a minute to look out over Many Glacier Valley and note the beige and gold rock before walking the 240 feet through the tunnel. The Belly River Valley heading north is starkly different, with red argillite striations that

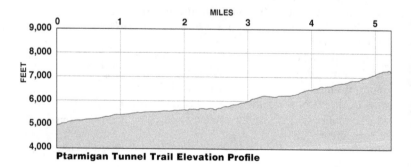

Ptarmigan Tunnel Trail Elevation Profile

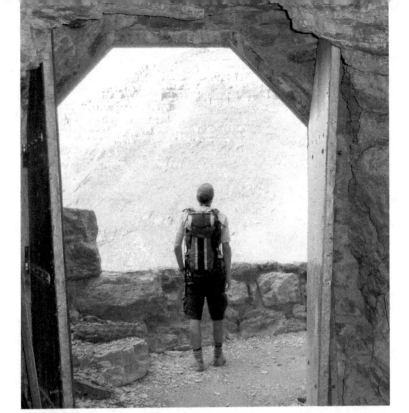

Ptarmigan Tunnel, *240 feet under a mountain pass, was built in 1930 to accommodate horses and pack trains. Today, humans and wildlife, including grizzly bears, use the tunnel, so look before heading into the rock-walled passageway.*

contrast with the thick, buff-colored limestone of the Siyeh Formation. It's worth a brief hike farther to see the Old Sun Glacier on 10,004-foot Mount Merritt to the west, tucked around Ptarmigan Wall and above Helen Lake. The man-made rock

 Geologic Interest

 OPTIONS

The hike is part of a popular two- to four-day backpack trip from Many Glacier to Ptarmigan Tunnel. You camp (permit required) at Elizabeth, Helen, and Poia Lakes; climb out of the Belly River Valley over Red Gap Pass; and finish at the Many Glacier Entrance Station—or hike farther into Many Glacier to Apikuni Trailhead or even on to Iceberg Lake Trailhead.

The 240-foot Ptarmigan Tunnel was blasted through the pass's rock in 1930 by the Civilian Conservation Corps so that horses and riders could travel from Many Glacier through the pass's tunnel and on to the Belly River drainage and Elizabeth, Helen, and Poia Lakes and back.

wall on the north side of the tunnel resembles the rock works along Going-to-the-Sun Road, providing a modicum of safety along an otherwise very exposed mountain pass.

Keep an eye on the weather, and remember that, in the same day, temperatures can vary from baking hot to blowing cold with pelting hail, lightning strikes, and 50-mile-per-hour wind gusts—summer in the mountains.

The tunnel is closed and locked October through early July because of snow. When the tunnel first opened in 1931, winter storms packed it with so much snow and ice that the tunnel often didn't melt out until late summer the next year. Steel doors were fitted to each side of the tunnel in 1975.

🚶 MILESTONES

▶1	0.0	Start at the Swiftcurrent Motor Inn parking area for cabins and Iceberg Lake Trailhead.
▶2	0.24	The trail meets the spur trail from Many Glacier Hotel; turn left/west.
▶3	1.0	Natural benches of red rock provide an amphitheater. Look closely to see wavy designs in the red and green argillite, from ancient waves in a Precambrian-age sea.
▶4	2.0	Look west to see Swiftcurrent Glacier.
▶5	2.38	A spur trail on the right leads to the outhouse a few steps off the main trail.
▶6	2.58	Ptarmigan Falls and footbridge
▶7	2.66	Junction with Ptarmigan Trail and the route to Ptarmigan Tunnel
▶8	4.32	Ptarmigan Lake
▶9	5.24	Ptarmigan Tunnel
▶10	5.25	Views of Old Sun Glacier, Elizabeth Lake, and the Belly River drainage. Return to trailhead.

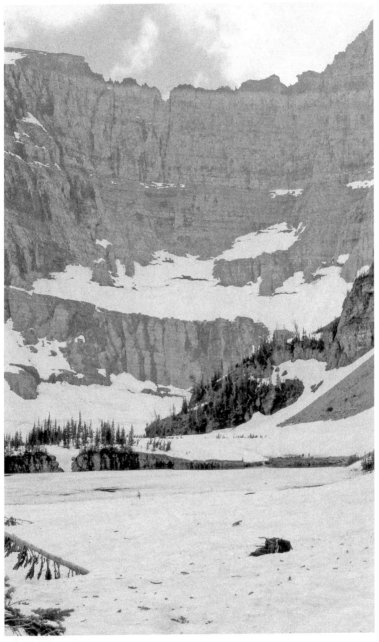

Iceberg Lake *is usually frozen over until mid-July, when icebergs float on the lake surface.*

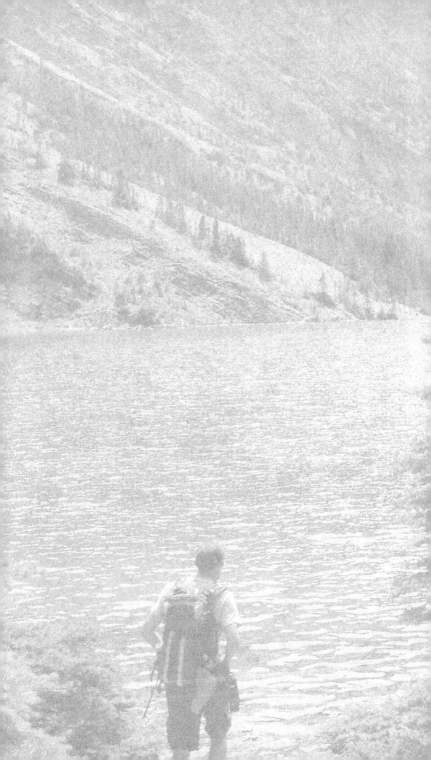

Waterton Lakes National Park, Canada

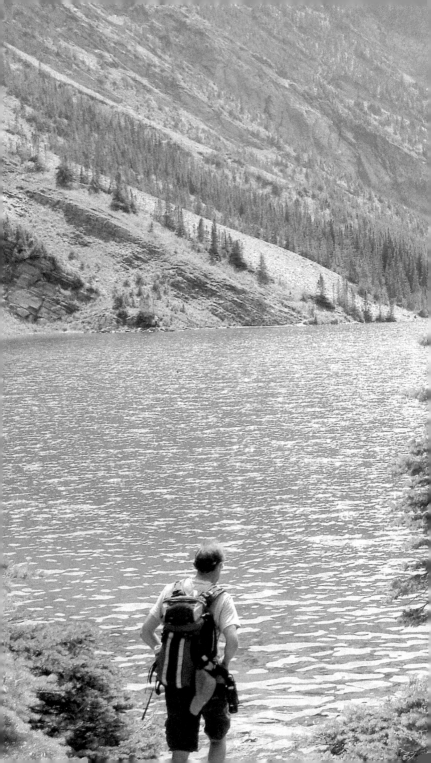

Waterton Lakes National Park, Canada

Waterton Lakes, the smaller 124,788-acre sister park to Glacier, still has impressive statistics: The two parks constitute the first International Peace Park, and both have significant and abundant flora and fauna that led to the distinction as a UNESCO World Heritage Site of special cultural and physical significance. Together, the parks encompass 1,720 square miles of mostly wild lands. Here, too, is a collision of mountains and prairie, where distinct alpine flora abruptly gives way to a prairie-grasslands ecosystem. The landscape was shaped by glaciers and ice sheets that formed over inland seas as the region cooled to an ice age, then again warmed to reveal sediments from an ancient sea from 1,500 million years ago. Visible today are seabed ripple marks, now fossilized among the layers of exposed rock. The mountains of Waterton are the result of crushing continental plates, which pushed the mountains into what's known today as the Lewis Overthrust of the Canadian Rockies. The sparkling lakes, which freeze over each winter, are the result of glaciation, as visitors see in the valleys of Upper Waterton and Akamina Lakes, and in the cirques, such as the one that encases Cameron Lake.

Waterton Township has visitor services, camping, and lodging properties, including the Prince of Wales Hotel that prominently perches atop what geologists call a "kame" (a big hill of deposited layers of gravel and sand from retreating glaciers). The deep lake encourages boating and swimming, although the water is generally very cold, even in August. Tour boats transport hikers and sightseers to trailheads, including to Crypt Lake Trail and Goat Haunt Ranger Station in the U.S., departure points for hikes mentioned in the West Side Trails chapter. Visitors who intend to take the boat to Goat Haunt and hike farther into Glacier must carry a passport, have backcountry camping permits, and carry food and gear for a few days in the mountains.

Overleaf and opposite: *Bertha Lake is a popular fishing, picnicking, and camping spot, plus dogs are allowed on this trail—a rarity.*

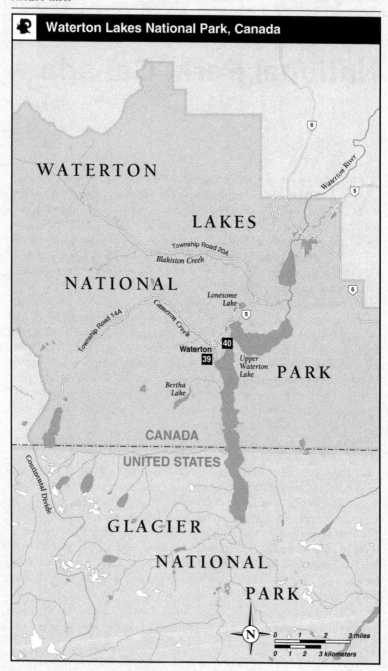

Waterton Lakes National Park, Canada

WATERTON

LAKES

NATIONAL

PARK

Township Road 20A

Blakiston Creek

Cameron Creek

Township Road 14A

Lonesome
Lake

Waterton River

Waterton

Bertha
Lake

Upper
Waterton
Lake

CANADA

UNITED STATES

Continental Divide

GLACIER

NATIONAL

PARK

N

0   1   2   3 miles

0   1   2   3 kilometers

TRAIL FEATURES TABLE

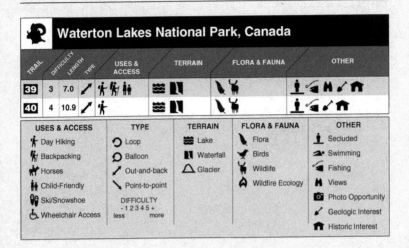

Waterton Lakes National Park, Canada

TRAIL	DIFFICULTY	LENGTH	TYPE	USES & ACCESS	TERRAIN	FLORA & FAUNA	OTHER
39	3	7.0	↗	🚶 🎒 👨‍👧	〰 ◗	❦ 🦌	⚲ 🎣 H ✎ ⌂
40	4	10.9	↗	🚶	〰 ◗	❦ 🦌	⚲ 🎣 ✎ ⌂

USES & ACCESS	TYPE	TERRAIN	FLORA & FAUNA	OTHER
🚶 Day Hiking	↺ Loop	〰 Lake	❦ Flora	⚲ Secluded
🎒 Backpacking	⊙ Balloon	◗ Waterfall	🦃 Birds	➘ Swimming
🐴 Horses	↗ Out-and-back	△ Glacier	🦌 Wildlife	🎣 Fishing
👨‍👧 Child-Friendly	＼ Point-to-point		🔥 Wildfire Ecology	H Views
🎿 Ski/Snowshoe	DIFFICULTY			📷 Photo Opportunity
♿ Wheelchair Access	- 1 2 3 4 5 + less more			✎ Geologic Interest
				⌂ Historic Interest

Hikers are often surprised by the fact that dogs are welcome in the Waterton Lakes backcountry and that, on some trails, bicycles are encouraged too—visitors should check locally for pet and bicycle rules and regulations.

Permits and Maps

Permits are not required for day hiking and biking in Waterton; however, backcountry permits are required for the nine wilderness campgrounds in the park and are available through the Waterton Lakes Information Centre. A national park fishing license is required for Waterton and can be purchased for one day or for the year at the park Information Centre.

Waterton Lakes National Park, Canada

TRAIL 39

Many hikers on the Bertha Lake Trail enjoy the trailside benches and picnicking at Lower Bertha Falls, yet the 21 switchbacks to reach Bertha Lake provide visitors with Upper Waterton Lake views, waterfalls, and craggy peaks, and make it one of the most popular hikes in Waterton.

Day hiking, backpacking, youth-friendly
7.0 miles
Out-and-back
Difficulty 1 2 **3** 4 5

TRAIL 40

Few places in the Northern Rockies offer naturally occurring tunnels, such as this one carved out of the rock by erosion near the upper reaches of the Crypt Lake Trail and only a few minutes before reaching the crystalline waters of the lake. Crypt Lake's shores are in both Canada and the U.S. but are only accessible by trail from Upper Waterton Lake.

Day hiking
10.9 miles
Out-and-back
Difficulty 1 2 3 **4** 5

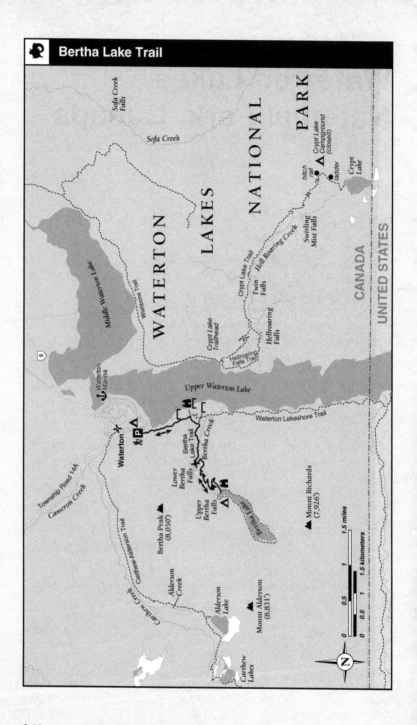

Sofa Creek Falls

Sofa Creek

PARK

NATIONAL

Crypt Lake Campground (closed)

hitch rail

ladder

Crypt Lake

Crypt Lake Trail

Swirling Mist Falls

Hell Roaring Creek

Twin Falls

LAKES

WATERTON

Crypt Lake Trailhead

Hellroaring Falls

Hellroaring Falls Trail

Middle Waterton Lake

Wishbone Trail

CANADA

UNITED STATES

5

Waterton Marina

Upper Waterton Lake

Waterton Lakeshore Trail

Waterton

Bertha Lake Trail

Bertha Creek

Lower Bertha Falls

Upper Bertha Falls

Bertha Lake

Mount Richards (7,926)

Township Road 14A

Cameron Creek

Bertha Peak (8,050)

Carthew-Alderson Trail

Alderson Creek

Carthew Creek

Alderson Lake

Mount Alderson (8,831)

Carthew Lakes

0   0.5   1   1.5 miles

0   0.5   1   1.5 kilometers

N

Bertha Lake Trail

Lake views, waterfalls, craggy peaks, and 21 switch-backs to reach Bertha Lake make this a challenging yet rewarding trail and one of the best in Waterton. Despite the vertical, many families and elders travel the well-maintained route to Bertha Falls and beyond—the steeper incline—to Bertha Lake. Parks Canada has thoughtfully provided benches along the wide route to the falls. Dogs (on leashes) are allowed on the trails in Waterton.

Best Time

The lower portion of the trail to the falls is snow-free by late May or early June; the entire route becomes snow-free by late June and is accessible through early October. Since portions of the trail are under direct sun, it's best to begin this climbing hike in the morning on hot summer days.

Finding the Trail

From Waterton Township, the trail begins from a well-marked parking area on Evergreen Avenue, two blocks south of Cameron Falls on the west side of Ruisseau Cameron Creek and west of Townsite Campground. The route follows the Waterton Lakeshore Trail 0.9 mile to the junction with Bertha Lake Trail.

TRAIL USE
Day hiking, backpack-ing, youth-friendly

LENGTH
7.0 miles, 3–6 hours; add 2.5 miles and 1–2 hours if you circumnavi-gate the lake

VERTICAL FEET
±1,509'

DIFFICULTY
1 2 **3** 4 5

TRAIL TYPE
Out-and-back

SURFACE TYPE
Dirt and gravel

START & END
N49° 02.816'
W113° 55.023'

FEATURES
Flora
Secluded
Geologic Interest
Historic Interest
Wildlife, Waterfalls
Lake, Fishing, Views

FACILITIES
Ranger station
Lodging, Restaurants
Stores, Gas
Guide services
Interpretive center
Campgrounds, Pit toilet

Trail Description

Lake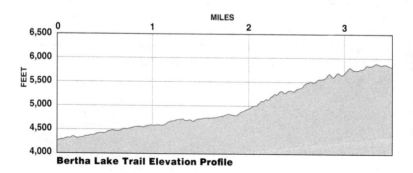

Initially, the trail parallels the 8-mile-long Upper Waterton Lake along the Waterton Lakeshore Trail, which leads to Goat Haunt Ranger Station inside Glacier National Park some 7 miles later. Spur trails allow spectacular views of Upper Waterton Lake and the surrounding peaks. At 0.9 miles, the route up to Lower and Upper Bertha Falls and the lake departs to the right/west and soon begins climbing alongside Bertha Creek, where several small cascades rush down the mountains.

Views

At 1.7 miles, Lower Bertha Falls sprays mist over the substantial footbridge that crosses just below the falls. Many hikers turn around here. Despite the switchbacks to come, what follows is a photogenic Rocky Mountain scene: a bigger waterfall, shaded trail, and crystalline lake.

Waterfall

At the sixth switchback is a remarkable tree with a huge U shape in the trunk, perfect for taking a break, as many hikers have done—the bark is rubbed to a shine from previous back pockets. After the 16th switchback, you will see the 200-foot Upper Bertha Falls. Bertha Lake is above that frothing cascade.

Waterfall

As you crest the last hill to the lake, there's a vantage point that reveals 7,926-foot Mount Richards,

Bertha Lake Trail Elevation Profile

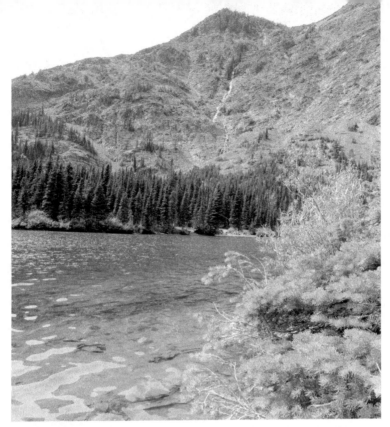

Bertha Lake Trail *begins gently and includes several park benches and viewpoints over Upper Waterton Lake before climbing 1,500 feet past waterfalls to the lake.*

8,831-foot Mount Alderson, and 8,050-foot Bertha Peak surrounding the 1.25- by 0.25-mile loch. Continue five minutes down to the shore, and you have choices: strip off boots and wade in; continue right/ northwest over a footbridge to the campsites and a lovely gravel beach; or go left/west around the lake

 Views

NOTES

Initially known as Spirit Lake, Bertha Lake, Creek, Falls, and Bay are named after a local homesteader who later went to jail for counterfeiting.

Lake to several beaches and fishing spots. A trail circumnavigates Bertha Lake, adding 2.5 miles to the hike.

Five campsites have raised, flat tent-site surfaces and are tucked away from the breezy lake, which means they can be buggy. The Waterton Township Campground at the trailhead has clean, hot, free showers; flat, grassy campsites near the lake; shelter trees; and nice dining buildings with tables, electricity, and woodstoves.

Camping ⚠

🚶 MILESTONES

►1	0.0	Start from the trailhead and parking area on Evergreen Street.
►2	0.5	The first of several trailside benches
►3	0.75	Waterton Lake overlook
►4	0.9	Junction with Bertha Lake trail; turn right/west.
►5	1.7	Lower Bertha Falls
►6	3.37	Upper Bertha Falls
►7	3.5	Bertha Lake. Return to trailhead.

A ranger-led evening program on bats and owls is worth an hour in the indoor amphitheater of the Townsite Campground.

Crypt Lake Trail

The route to Crypt Lake passes spectacular water-falls and a summer's worth of wildflowers as hikers climb past spent early bloomers at lower elevations and the same flowers in full bloom of August at higher elevations. Bears frequent the area and use the trail, as evidenced by trees with claw marks scarring the bark at different heights. The trees, now tagged by researchers with white or orange markers some 10 feet high, have strands of barbed wire attached to the bark to snag bear hair for research.

Best Time

The trail is best accessed from late June through early September, when the Waterton Shoreline Cruise Co. tour boat *Miss Waterton* offers shuttles from Waterton Marina to the trailhead. The fee includes round-trip transportation.

Finding the Trail

From the Watertown Marina, ride the *Miss Waterton* hiker shuttle, which departs at 9 a.m. and 10 a.m. each summer morning (**watertoncruise.com**). After the 15-minute ferry, the boat docks at the Crypt Lake Trailhead, immediately right/south of the dock and in the trees. The return boat shuttle leaves Crypt Lake Trailhead at 4 p.m. and 5:30 p.m. Don't miss the shuttle—the boat captain doesn't wait for tardy hikers.

TRAIL USE
Day hiking

LENGTH
10.9 miles, 5–8 hours
with boat shuttle

VERTICAL FEET
±2,130

DIFFICULTY
1 2 3 **4** 5

TRAIL TYPE
Out-and-back

SURFACE TYPE
Dirt, gravel, and rock

START & END
N49° 03.218'
W113° 54.412'

FEATURES
Flora
Secluded
Geologic Interest
Historic Interest
Wildlife
Waterfalls
Lake, Fishing

FACILITIES
Ranger station
Lodging, Restaurants
Stores, Gas
Interpretive center
Tour boat
Campgrounds
Guide service

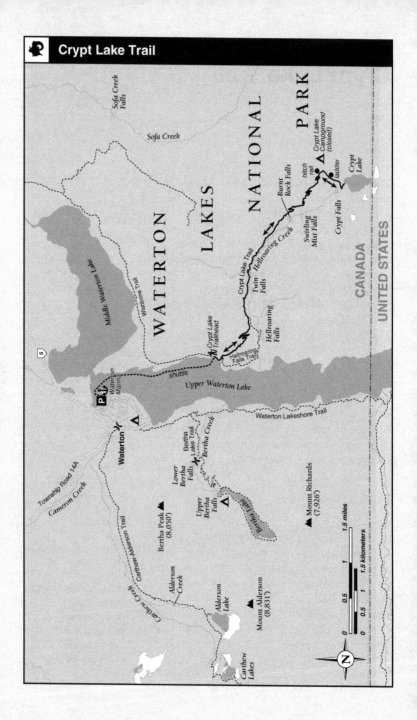

Crypt Lake Trail

WATERTON LAKES NATIONAL PARK

Sofa Creek Falls

Sofa Creek

Crypt Lake Campground (closed)

hitch rail

ladder

Crypt Lake

Burnt Rock Falls

Swirling Mist Falls

Crypt Falls

Crypt Lake Trail

Hellroaring Creek

Twin Falls

CANADA

UNITED STATES

Wishbone Trail

Middle Waterton Lake

Crypt Lake Trailhead

Hellroaring Falls

Hellroaring Falls Trail

5

Waterton Marina

shuttle

Upper Waterton Lake

P

Waterton

Waterton Lakeshore Trail

Bertha Lake Trail

Bertha Creek

Lower Bertha Falls

Upper Bertha Falls

Bertha Lake

Mount Richards (7,926)

Township Road 14A

Cameron Creek

Carthew-Alderson Trail

Bertha Peak (8,050)

Carthew Creek

Alderson Creek

Alderson Lake

Mount Alderson (8,831)

Carthew Lakes

1.5 miles

1.5 kilometers

0.5   1

0.5   1

0   N

Another option is the 6.8-mile Wishbone Trail; this trail is open to bicyclists and equestrians and begins along Chief Mountain Highway. Route finding is difficult and trail signs confusing or nonexistent in the final mile to the Crypt Lake Trailhead.

Trail Description

At 0.2 mile, the first waterfall, Hellroaring, is accessed via a 1.3-mile spur loop, which is steep and best reserved for the return hike. After the initial dozen switchbacks and the other end of the Hellroaring Falls spur at 1.4 miles, the trail cruises gently for 1.2 miles in the Hellroaring Creek Valley until the spruce and Douglas fir forest gives way to rocky and scree-filled alpine scenes and the second major water feature, Burnt Rock Falls. Here the trail switchbacks up 1,000 feet, along Vimy Ridge's skirt. South across Crypt Valley, the 500-foot Crypt Falls marks the destination—almost. Crypt Lake is cradled above and to the left of the falls, although not visible. Finally, and mercifully if it's hot, the trail slips back into trees—look for huckleberries here—and passes the former Crypt Campsite. There is still a pit toilet, which is more often than not stocked with toilet paper. The next quarter mile might unnerve hikers unaccustomed to exposure

 Waterfall

 Waterfall

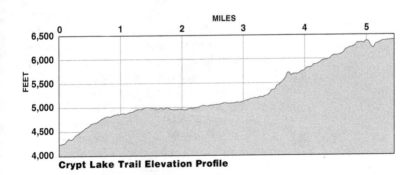

Crypt Lake Trail Elevation Profile

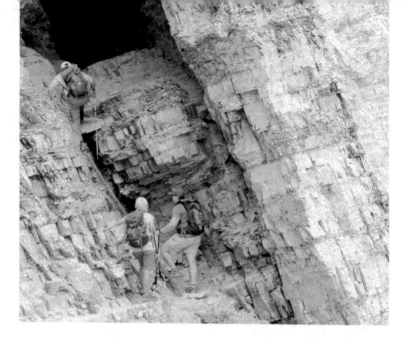

Crypt Lake's *50-foot-long natural tunnel leads to a crystalline lake that's back in the US.*

If you hike around Crypt Lake, you will walk along the international boundary, the longest undefended border in the world.

Waterfall

Lake

and the significant 500-foot drop below. Some hikers retreat here.

The natural tunnel, carved out of the rock by erosion, is just ahead. A metal ladder is secured to the rock ledge. Taller folks should remove backpacks before attempting the tunnel; it's a crab-crawl sideways scuttle for 50 feet before you pop out on the other side. Here's where the intimidating exposure begins. After a few tenuous steps along a rock ledge, hikers can grab a cable that is attached to the cliff—that's the route. Soon the trail is back on the forest path, where it sweeps near the top of Crypt Falls. A 40-foot spur edges up to the precipice. Walk upstream about 200 feet to the crypt, where water from the lake above has scoured an underground tunnel. Water splashes out of the rock here.

After another few minutes, hikers find the 0.35- by 0.25-mile lake, which edges into the U.S. The Wilson Mountain Range, part of the cirque surrounding emerald-green to turquoise-blue Crypt Lake, is nearly entirely inside Montana's Glacier National Park—no border patrol here, but there is a gentle trail around the lake that adds 0.65 mile to the hike. Crypt Lake has beaches, logs for benches, and refreshingly cool water for soaking toes. While the trail below has been filled with huckleberries, harebell, Oregon grape, thimbleberry, maple, and juniper in shaded spots, as well as cinquefoil, yarrow, and the rare alpine pygmy poppy, beware of the stinging nettle along the trail and the lakeshore.

Dogs are allowed both on this trail and on the tour boat; however, the upper half of the trail can be very hot, with few water crossings for canine trekkers. The trail from the former Crypt Lake Campsite to the tunnel crosses rocky ledges. The trail after the tunnel has quite significant exposure and difficult rock climbs where dog handlers may have to carry their furry charges—hiking with a dog past the old campsite is dangerous and not recommended.

Crypt Lake basin is an example of glacial melt, which formed the valleys and deep bowls for lakes 10,000 years ago.

 Flora

🚶 MILESTONES

►1	0.0	Start from the boat dock and ride the *Miss Waterton* tour boat.
►2	0.0	Disembark the tour boat and see the trailhead above the beach on the right/south.
►3	0.2	Junction with the Hellroaring Falls Trail
►4	1.3	Junction with the upper end of Hellroaring Falls Trail
►5	2.0	Falls view
►6	3.0	Falls view
►7	4.3	Pit toilet, hitching rail, and former campground
►8	5.0	Tunnel
►9	5.3	Crypt Creek above Crypt Falls
►10	5.45	Crypt Lake. Return to trailhead and boat dock.

Appendix 1

Top-Rated Trails

Appendix 2

Campgrounds and RV Parks

Glacier National Park

Glacier National Park's 13 campgrounds feature 1,009 sites. Most campgrounds in Glacier are first come, first served, except for Fish Creek, St. Mary, and half of the group sites in Apgar. These campsites can be reserved in advance at **recreation.gov.** Backcountry campsites can be reserved in person at the Backcountry Rangers' Office in Apgar or in advance via **nps.gov/glac** and then faxing a backcountry campsite application. Inside Glacier National Park, campground rates range from $10 to $23 per night. Only Apgar and Saint Mary Campgrounds remain open year-round, but they are considered primitive or winter camping, when no water is available.

Note that food-storage regulations are in effect year-round and demand that all food is securely stored at all times in a vehicle or in a hard-sided camping unit of solid, non-pliable material; suspended from any National Park Service–designated food hanging device; or secured inside an NPS-designated storage locker, in an Interagency Grizzly Bear Committee–approved, bear-resistant container, or inside a dwelling. Violation of food storage regulations may result in a $75 fine and fees and/or confiscation of improperly stored items.

The following are Glacier National Park's 13 campgrounds:

- Apgar
- Avalanche
- Bowman Lake
- Cut Bank
- Fish Creek
- Kintla Lake
- Logging Creek
- Many Glacier
- Quartz Creek
- Rising Sun
- Sprague Creek
- St. Mary
- Two Medicine

Commercial Campgrounds outside Glacier National Park

For more information on campgrounds outside Glacier, check out visitmt.com.

Eastside of Glacier
Glacier Meadow RV Park
406-226-4479; glaciermeadowrvpark.com

Sleeping Wolf Campground and RV Park
406-338-7207; blackfeetcountry.com/campgrounds

St. Mary Area
Chewing Blackbones Campground and RV Park
406-338-7406; blackfeetcountry.com/campgrounds

Duck Lake Lodge and Campground
406-338-5770 or 406-338-2777; ducklakelodge.com

Elkhorn Cabins & Campground
406-732-9293; elkhorncabinsandcampgrounds.com

Johnson's Campground & RV Park
406-732-4207; johnsonsofstmary.com

KOA
406-732-4122; koa.com or goglacier.com

Leaning Tree Campground & Café
406-338-5322

Red Eagle Motel & RV Park
406-732-4453; redeaglemotelrvpark.com

Westside of Glacier
Crooked Tree Motel & RV Park
406-387-5531; home.centurytel.net/~crookedt/

Glacier Campground
406-387-5689; glaciercampground.com

Glacier Haven RV and Campground
406-888-9987; glacierhavenrv-campground.com

Glacier Peaks RV
406-892-2133; glacierpeaksrvpark.com

San-Suz-Ed RV Park, Campground, and Bed-and-Breakfast
406-387-5280; sansuzedrvpark.com

Timber Wolf Resort
406-387-9653; timberwolfresort.com

Whitefish Bike Retreat
406-260-0274; **whitefishbikeretreat.com**

Whitefish KOA
406-862-4242; **glacierparkkoa.com**

Whitefish RV Park
406-862-7275; **whitefishrvpark.com**

Waterton Lakes National Park

The following three campgrounds are operated by Parks Canada:

- Townsite Campground
- Crandell Mountain Campground
- Belly River Campground

For more information, visit **pc.gc.ca** or call 403-859-5133.

The following two campgrounds are privately owned and near Waterton Lakes National Park:

Waterton Springs Campground
(bordering the park)
403-859-2247; **watertonspringscamping.com**

Crooked Creek Campground
(6 miles east of park entrance)
403-653-1100; **wnha.ca**

Flathead National Forest

There are 31 established campgrounds in the Flathead National Forest, many of which are near Glacier National Park and include:

- Glacier View Ranger District's Big Creek, Moose Lake, Red Meadow, and Tuchuck Campgrounds
- Hungry Horse Ranger District's Devil Creek Campground, Devil's Corkscrew Campground, Doris Creek Campground, Emery Bay Campground, Handkerchief Lake, Riverside Boating Site, Lakeview Campground, Lid Creek Campground, Lost Johnny Campground, Lost Johnny Point Campground, and Murray Bay Campground
- Spotted Bear Ranger District's Beaver Creek Campground, Peter's Creek Campground, and Spotted Bear Campground.

For more information on these campgrounds, visit **www.fs.usda.gov/flathead.**

Lewis and Clark National Forest

Summit Campground near East Glacier
www.fs.usda.gov/lcnf

Appendix 3

Hotels, Lodges, Motels, and Resorts

Montana's remote and rugged lands dominate the landscape of the country's fourth largest state at 147,046 square miles. During the last ice age, 10,000 to 14,000 years ago, western Montana's valleys slumbered under a massive sheet of glacial ice. Glacially carved valleys, now rich in topsoils and wildlife, clean lakes and plentiful waterfowl, accommodated American Indians for the past 10,000–12,000 years, and those sculpted valleys became the namesake for Glacier National Park. By the time the Corps of Discovery ventured near Glacier in 1805, while exploring the 1803 Louisiana Purchase, American Indians camped, fished, and hunted with great success—yet did not reveal the low-elevation mountain pass to the Lewis and Clark expedition; thus, the great Glacier ecosystem wasn't developed by European descendants until the past century.

Travelers find the great lodges of Glacier and Waterton Lakes National Parks awe-inspiring for lodging, as well as a day's visit for dining or just an ice-cream cone and photographs. An array of lodging options in and around the parks varies from primitive tent camping to mom-and-pop motels, bed-and-breakfasts, and upscale ranch-resorts. A nearly complete list of camping and lodging facilities inside and nearby Glacier and Waterton can be found on Montana's official state travel site, **visitmt.com.**

This appendix includes general comments about each area of and near the parks.

Westside of Glacier National Park and the Flathead Valley

The tiny berg at the western entrance to Glacier National Park, West Glacier, has a handful of hotels, motels, campgrounds, and eateries, some of which are only open during the summer. Since West Glacier is an Amtrak stop, it's nice to know that many lodging properties are within walking distance of the station. The remote and fantastically beautiful Polebridge, Montana, area is known for the eclectic **North Fork Hostel** (nfhostel.com), **The Way Less Traveled Bed and Breakfast** (thewaylesstraveled.com), a few campgrounds, and U.S. Forest Service rental cabins (**recreation.gov**; search using ZIP Code 59928). The tourism region, Glacier Country, Montana, offers significant information on lodging and tourism at **glaciermt.com.** The resort community of Whitefish (**explorewhitefish.com**) is known for year-round recreation, lodging, and eateries on Whitefish Lake and at the base of Whitefish Mountain Ski Resort. Kalispell, the county seat and landing strip for Glacier International Airport, provides all amenities for a Montana visit and is a jumping-off point to other Flathead Valley communities, such as Bigfork and Polson, both on Flathead Lake, and Whitefish, Columbia Falls, West Glacier, Polebridge, Essex, East Glacier, and on to Waterton, Canada.

The Lodges of Glacier National Park and Waterton Lakes National Park

Glacier's nine lodges, motor inns, and chalets and 13 campgrounds are managed by a variety of organizations. Glacier Park Lodges/Xanterra Parks & Resorts (**glaciernationalparklodges.com**) operates the **Village Inn Motel, Lake McDonald Lodge, Rising Sun Motor Inn, Swiftcurrent Motor Inn,** and **Many Glacier Hotel,** all inside the park. **Apgar Village Lodge** (westglacier.com/apgar_village_lodge .php) features 28 rustic cabins and 20 lakeside motel units on Lake McDonald at Apgar Village. **Granite Park and Sperry Chalets,** the two backcountry chalets, are operated by Belton Chalets, Inc. (**granite parkchalet.com**) and are accessible only by hiking trail or horseback ride. Five full-service properties are managed by Glacier Park Inc. (**glacierparkinc.com**) and include **Motel Lake McDonald** on Lake McDonald, **Prince of Wales Hotel** in Waterton, **Glacier Park Lodge** in East Glacier, **Grouse Mountain Lodge** in Whitefish, and **St. Mary Lodge, Cabins, and Motel** in St. Mary. **Belton Chalet,** just outside the West Glacier entrance, offers year-round lodging and dining at the historic inn (**beltonchalet.com**). **Izzak Walton Inn,** on Glacier's southern edge, is open year-round for hikers and skiers and is a whistle stop along the Amtrak line (**izaakwaltoninn.com**).

East Side of Glacier National Park

The East Glacier area (**eastglacierpark.info**) has a handful of mom-and-pop motels, cabins, hostels, and lodges, many of which are within walking distance of the Amtrak station and Glacier Park Lodge at the intersection of US 2 and MT 49. The tourism region, Russell Country (**russellcountry.com**), lists lodging and recreation opportunities in the

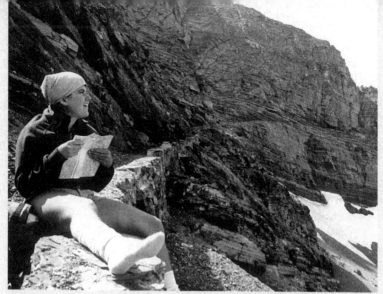

Ptarmigan Tunnel Trail *connects the Many Glacier Valley with the Belly River drainage and includes a man-made rock wall on the north side of the tunnel along the trail above Elizabeth Lake.*

gateway communities south and east of Glacier, including Great Falls, Montana, and its Great Falls International Airport.

Waterton Lakes National Park and Townsite

The tiny community of Waterton in Alberta, Canada, has a handful of lodging properties and an extensive campground, mostly open summers only. Parks Canada lists facilities on its website (**pc.gc.ca**), and visitors will also find useful information on the local Waterton website (**my waterton.ca**). The **Prince of Wales Hotel,** managed by Glacier Park Inc. (**glacierparkinc.com**), is open summers only.

Appendix 4

Major Organizations

Glacier National Park Conservancy
402 Ninth St. W
Columbia Falls, MT 59912
406-892-3250; **glacierconservancy.org**

Glacier Institute
PO Box 1887
Kalispell, MT 59903
406-755-1211; **glacierinstitute.org**

Crown of the Continent Research Learning Center
nps.gov/glac/naturescience/ccrlc.htm

Roundtable on the Crown of the Continent
crownroundtable.org

Coalition to Protect the Rocky Mountain Front
406-466-2600; **savethefront.org**

Flathead National Forest Supervisor's Office
650 Wolfpack Way
Kalispell, MT 59901
406-758-5208; **www.fs.usda.gov/flathead**

Flathead Avalanche Center
650 Wolfpack Way
Kalispell, MT 59901
Avalanche Advisory Hot Line: 406-257-8402; Office: 406-261-9873
flatheadavalanche.org

National Parks Conservation Association
777 Sixth St. NW, Suite 700
Washington, D.C. 20001-3723
800-628-7275; **npca.org**

Montana Chapter of the Sierra Club
PO Box 1290
Bozeman, MT 59771
406-582-8365; **montana.sierraclub.org**

The Nature Conservancy's Pine Butte Guest Ranch
351 South Fork Rd.
Choteau, MT 59422
406-466-2158; **pinebutteguestranch.com**

Glacier Natural History Association Bookstore
12544 US 2
West Glacier, MT 59936
406-888-5756

North Fork Preservation Association
gravel.org

Montana Wilderness Association
Whitefish Field Office
750 Second St. W, Suite A
Whitefish, MT 59937
406-730-2006; **wildmontana.org**

Blackfeet Nation
tribalnations.mt.gov/blackfeet.asp

Confederated Salish and Kootenai Tribes
cskt.org

Ktunaxa Nation
ktunaxa.org

Sierra Club BC
301–2994 Douglas St.
Victoria, BC, Canada V8T 4N4
250-386-5255; **sierraclub.bc.ca/our-work/flathead**

Canadian Parks and Wilderness Society
British Columbia Chapter
410–698 Seymour St.
Vancouver, BC, Canada V6B 3K6
604-685-7445; **cpawsbc.org**

Wildsight Canada
2–495 Wallinger Ave.
Kimberley, BC, Canada V1A 1Z6
250-427-9325; **wildsight.ca**

Appendix 5

Useful Books

Note: Most of the books listed below are available through the non-profit Glacier Conservancy and at **glacierconservancy.org.**

Backpacking and Hiking Books and Maps

Beffort, Brian. *Joy of Backpacking.* Berkeley, CA: Wilderness Press, 2007.

Schneider, Bill and Russ, eds. *Backpacking Tips: Trail-tested Wisdom from FalconGuide Authors, 2nd ed.* Guilford, CT: Falcon Publishing, 2005.

Trails Illustrated Map: North Fork #313. Evergreen, CO: National Geographic Maps, 2009.

Trails Illustrated Map: Many Glacier #314. Evergreen, CO: National Geographic Maps, 2009.

Trails Illustrated Map: Two Medicine #315. Evergreen, CO: National Geographic Maps, 2009.

Trails Illustrated Map: Glacier/Waterton Lakes National Parks #215. Evergreen, CO: National Geographic Maps, 2004.

Glacier National Park 7.5-minute topographic maps. Reston, VA: U.S. Geological Survey, 2011.

Guidebooks

Arthur, Jean. *Winter Trails Montana: The Best Cross-Country Ski & Snowshoe Trails.* Guilford, CT: Globe Pequot, 2000.

Holterman, Jack. *Place Names of Glacier National Park, 3rd ed.* Helena, MT: Riverbend Publishing, 2006.

Lomax, Becky. *Moon Glacier National Park.* Berkeley, CA: Moon Handbooks, 2013.

Nystrom, Andrew and Morgan Konn. *Top Trails Yellowstone & Grand Teton National Parks, 2nd ed.* Berkeley, CA: Wilderness Press, 2009.

Raup, Omar. *Geology Along Going-to-the-Sun Road.* Guilford, CT: Glacier Natural History Association and Falcon Publishing, 1983.

Shea, David. *Animal Tracks of Glacier National Park.* West Glacier, MT: Glacier Natural History Association, 1986.

History and Literature

Arthur, Jean. *Hellroaring: Fifty Years on The Big Mountain.* Golden, CO: Whitefish Editions, 1996.

Fraley, John. *A Woman's Way West: In and Around Glacier National Park from 1925 to 1990.* Libby, MT: Big Mountain Publishing, 1998.

Guthrie, C.W. *All Aboard! For Glacier.* Helena, MT: Farcountry Press, 2004.

Lawrence, Tom. *Pictures, a Park, and a Pulitzer: Mel Ruder and the Hungry Horse News.* Helena, MT: Farcountry Press, 2003.

Linderman, Frank B. *Indian Old-Man Stories: More Sparks from War Eagle's Lodge-Fire.* Cartwright Press, reprinted 2011.

Moylan, Bridget. *Glacier's Grandest: A Pictorial History of the Hotels and Chalets of Glacier National Park.* Missoula, MT: Pictorial Histories Publishing Co., 1994.

Wissler, Clark and D.C. Duball. *Mythology of the Blackfoot Indians, 2nd ed.* Lincoln, NE: University of Nebraska Press, 2007.

Natural History

Fisher, Chris C. *Birds of the Rocky Mountains.* Edmonton, Alberta, Canada: Lone Pine Publishing, 1997.

Kimball, Shannon Fitzpatrick and Peter Lesica. *Wildflowers of Glacier National Park and Surrounding Areas.* Missoula, MT: Mountain Press Publishing, 2010.

Harada, Sumio and Kathleen Yale. *Mountain Goats of Glacier National Park.* Helena, MT: Farcountry Press, 2008.

Herrero, Stephen. *Bear Attacks.* Guilford, CT: Lyons Press, 2002.

Rockwell, David. *Glacier: A Natural History Guide.* Guilford, CT: Falcon Publishing, 2007.

Schneider, Bill. *Bear Aware, 3rd ed.* Guilford, CT: FalconGuides, 2004.

Schneider, Russ. *Fishing Glacier National Park, 2nd ed.* Guilford, CT: FalconGuides, 2002.

Waldt, Ralph. *Crown of the Continent.* Helena, MT: Riverbend Publishing, 2008.

Index

N

national parks, research in, 3
navigating trail entries, xv–xvi
navigation devices, 17–18
Nicholson, Jack, 166
Night of the Grizzlies incident, 131, 135–136
Night of the Grizzlies (Olsen), 136
Niitsitapi people, 3
North Fork, Flathead River, 81, 85
North Fork trails. *See* West Side trails
northern bog lemming, 8
Northern Piikani Indians, 4
Numa Ridge, 85

O

Oldman Lake, 201
Old Person, Chief Earl, 211
Old Sun Glacier, 257
organizations, major, 285–286
Otokomi Lake/Rose Creek Trail, 121, 167–171
Otokomi Mountain, 167

P

Paddlefish Sports, 13
Painted Tepee, 205
Pat's Gas & Cycle Rental, 13
Peacock, Doug, 75
permits, camping, fees, 11
phones, 18
Piegan Glacier, 149
Piegan Indians, 151
Piegan Mountain, 129, 139, 149, 150
Piegan Pass Trail, 119, 147–151, 159
pink bitterroot flower, 181
pink snow, 100
Pitamakan (Blackfeet woman), 202
Pitamakan Pass Trail, 197–201
Polebridge, Montana, 23
Pray Lake, 201
Preston Park, 144, 146
Prince of Wales Hotel, 263
Ptarmigan Lake, 256
Ptarmigan Tunnel Trail, 233, 254–259
Ptarmigan Wall, 251
Pumpelly Pillar, 194

Q

Quarter Circle Bridge, 69, 71
Quartz Lake Loop, 30, 88–92

R

Red Bench Fire of 1988, 92
Red Eagle Fire of 2006, 174
Red Eagle Lake, 166, 174, 175
Red Eagle Lake Trail, 173
Red Eagle Mountain, 175
regions, navigating, xiv–xv
renting boats, 13
research in national parks, 3
reserving campsites, 279
resorts, 282–284
Reuter Peak, 85
Reynolds Creek, 159
Reynolds Creek Campground, 154
Reynolds Mountain, 123
Richardson ground squirrel, 8
Rising Sun Boat Dock, 164, 165
Rising Sun Campground, 113
Rising Sun Motor Inn, 163
Rising Wolf Mountain, 189, 201
Roberts Fire of 2003, 70, 80
Rockwell Falls, 205
Rose, Charlie Otokomi, 170
Running Eagle Falls Nature Trail, 186, 188–191
RV parks
    Glacier National Park, 279–281
    Waterton Lakes National Park, Canada, 281

S

Sacred Dancing Cascade, 63
safety around bears, 6, 7, 13, 113
Saint Mary area
    See also Logan Pass and Saint Mary area
    map, 114
Saint Mary Campground, 113
Saint Mary Falls, 160, 164, 165
Saint Mary Falls Trail with Virginia Falls, Baring Falls, 120, 162–166
Saint Mary Lake, 161, 163, 166
Saint Mary Lodge, 173
Saint Mary River, 154
Salamander Glacier, 235, 245

About the Author

Jean Arthur

Jean Arthur has hiked, backpacked, skied, biked, boated, and floated Montana's trails, slopes, rivers, and lakes for 35 years. As a teenager, she

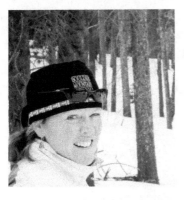

began writing for her high school newspaper, which led to a journalism degree from the University of Oregon and a Masters of Fine Art in fiction writing from the University of Montana. Jean has taught writing at Montana State University since 2003.

Jean has authored four books, including: *Hellroaring: Fifty Years on The Big Mountain; Timberline and a Century of Skiing Mount Hood; Winter Trails Montana: The Best Cross-Country Ski & Snowshoe Trails;* and now *Top Trails Glacier National Park.* She has contributed chapters to four books on outdoor adventuring, and her writing frequents the pages of Alaska Air's in-flight magazine, Horizon Air's in-flight magazine, *Ski Trax* magazine, Vacations Publications, and many other adventure and travel publications.

Series Creator

Joe Walowski conceived of the Top Trails series in 2003 and was series editor of the first three titles: *Top Trails Los Angeles, Top Trails San Francisco Bay Area,* and *Top Trails Lake Tahoe.* He lives in Seattle.

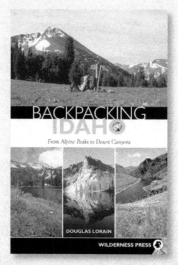

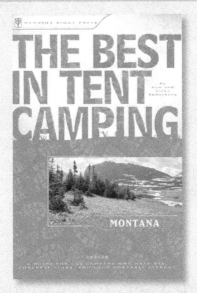

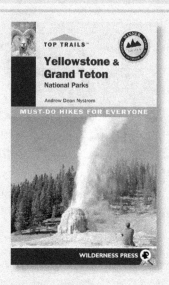